What's the Remedy for That?

The Definitive Homeopathy Guide
to Mastering Everyday
Self-Care Without Drugs

Kathleen K. Fry, MD, CTHHom

Collette Avenue Press

Printed in the United States of America

First Printing: March 2017

ISBN 978-0-9847534-2-0
Collette Avenue Press

Dedication

To my parents Dick Kolt and Betty Atchison Kolt
who raised five healthy children
and to my siblings Betsy, Richard, Don & Bob
who helped them do it.

Thank You

Thank you so much for buying my book.
I hope you will enjoy exploring the healing
art of homeopathy and dipping your
toes into the waters of self healing.

As a special thank you,
I am offering a BONUS GIFT
of my free report entitled
"The Top Ten Remedies to
Never Travel Without."

It's an annotated guide of the most
important remedies to have when you
are away from home, complete with
instructions on how to use them.

Just go to my website at
DrKathiFry.com and click on the
Remedies for Travel button
to download your free copy.

Thank you!
Dr. Kathi Fry

Contents

Contents

Acknowledgments

As with any project, it takes a village and I am blessed to live among some of the most helpful people in any village.

Betsy Kolt whose keen eye for design produced a wonderful cover. Heidi Grauel for her editing talents; she made it all seem very easy. Deana Riddle for her help with the cover and her advice on all things bookish.

Martha Bullen, whose knowledge of the publishing world has been invaluable in helping this book get out into the world.

My Quantum Leap mastermind group coaches and fellow creators: Geoffrey Berwind, Judy Cohen, Brenda Reynolds, Carol Clifton, and Sharon Cluck. What a blessing to have such happy companions on this creative journey.

And last but not least, I want to say a special thanks to Steve Harrison and all the wonderful people at Quantum Leap. Steve has a special skill of recruiting and mentoring talented people who love helping others to fulfill their missions. I have learned so much from all of them and I'm grateful to my friend John Vnuk for introducing me to the Quantum Leap program. It has been a life changer for me and I'm very grateful.

Preface

Your body is a miracle. You are made up of trillions of little energetic beings (i.e., cells) that perform thousands and thousands of intricate functions all day, all night, around the clock, without you having to even think about it! As you are reading this, your gut is digesting your last meal and your bone marrow is making red blood cells that will last exactly 120 days. Your nervous system is a beautiful symphony of neurons firing in such perfect harmony that you can read this page and understand what the words on it mean while your lungs breathe and your heart beats—all without your conscious control.

No matter what medical diagnosis you may have been given, or what physical condition may be afflicting you, the parts of your body that are working well outnumber those that are not—right up until the moment of your death. At any given moment, well-being is your dominant, natural state because this is how you were created. You started from the union of two cells, one from your mother and one from your father. Once those two cells united, they began to divide and multiply, growing first into a tube that would become your nervous system. With each cell division, those cells differentiated into all the tissues that would become, in the vast majority of cases, the perfect baby whose 10 fingers and 10 toes your parents lovingly counted at the moment of your birth.

Since that miraculous moment of your birth, your body has continued to grow hair and fingernails, digest millions of molecules of food, breathe in innumerable atoms of air and tirelessly pump liters of blood nonstop without any thinking or planning required from you.

This is the beauty of who you are as a human being. That beautiful orchestra that is your body is under the control of the Vital Force, an energetic powerhouse of well-being. Every cell in every tissue of your body is kept in alignment with the Source that set it all in motion the moment those two cells from your parents met.

When we are sick, we often forget what it feels like to be well, especially if we have been suffering for a long time. There is a spiritual teaching that states, "What you focus on, expands." So, my advice to you and to all my patients is to remind yourself every day that no matter what symptoms you may currently have, focus on the innate well-being that is your natural state.

You have a dynamic, powerful force inside you that is constantly striving to make you thrive. When that force gets weakened, your body produces symptoms. Paying attention to those symptoms and understanding what the Vital Force is "asking" for in the way of help is the key to restoring your body to its natural state of vitality. For me, this is the blessing of the art and science of homeopathy. Using substances from nature prepared to enhance the vibrational power inherent in everything God created, it is possible to restore and maintain the natural state of health and well-being that is our birthright.

Introduction

What if, instead of an expensive and time-consuming visit to the ER, you could safely and effectively treat yourself and your family at home for common ailments such as colds, flu, ear infections, and even food poisoning?

It's completely possible with time and doctor-tested homeopathic remedies, most of which are readily available in your local health food store. In my first book, *VITALITY! How to Get It and Keep It: A Homeopath's Guide to Vibrant Health Without Drugs*, I discussed the origin and history of homeopathic medicine, case histories from my own practice, and a section on how to use the most common remedies available over the counter.

This book is designed to give you more detailed information on the most common remedies for the most common ailments that afflict most everyone at some time in their lives. Who hasn't occasionally suffered with a horrible cold or a bad case of the flu while traveling? Nothing can ruin a vacation or a business trip more than being stuck in a hotel room away from home, puking your guts out!

But if you have the right knowledge of how to safely and effectively use these simple but powerful remedies, you can avoid costly trips to the ER, treat yourself when traveling, and shorten the time of an acute illness, all without pharmaceutical drugs.

For more than 25 years, I have been teaching my patients and clients how to use these remedies for everything from ear infections and fever to toothaches and altitude sickness. In this straightforward book, you too can benefit from my years of experience and learn how to use these remedies with confidence.

I am often asked, "How is homeopathy different from conventional, herbal, or naturopathic medicine?" In a nutshell (a rather large one), homeopathy is a form of alternative, vibrational healing that stimulates the body's ability to heal itself without drugs by strengthening the Vital Force. The Vital Force is the unseen, energetic power that guides every physiologic function of living beings.

The principles of homeopathy were discovered and codified by Dr. Samuel Hahnemann, a physician who lived and worked in Germany at the end of the 18th century. In those days, what passed for conventional medicine included such brutal treatments as bloodletting and inducing vomiting, sweating, and purging with caustic compounds like arsenic and mercury. Dr. Hahnemann became disillusioned with such cures that were worse than the disease. So, he gave up the practice of medicine and supported his family by translating ancient medical texts from their original Greek and Latin into German. Through his studies of the writings of Hippocrates, Galen, and Paracelsus, he discovered the underlying principle *Similia similibus curentur* which is Latin for "likes are cured by likes." This means that a substance given to healthy people induces a set of symptoms in a process called a proving. When that same set of symptoms is recognized in a sick person, that substance can be used to heal the illness.

The purpose of homeopathic treatment of any condition is to help the Vital Force achieve a state of optimal health. This healthy state is reflected in the absence of disease symptoms. All symptoms are just a message from the Vital Force indicating a need for help. Thus, headaches serve a purpose. Determining which remedy the Vital Force is requesting and then taking that remedy for as long as needed forms the basis of treatment.

By removing the root cause of headaches, or any other condition, homeopathic remedies can successfully and permanently restore a person to health. Once this state of health is achieved, there is no longer a need to take a remedy unless a new set of symptoms develops. It is possible to stop the cycle of suffering and obviate the need to take pharmaceutical drugs or even homeopathic remedies over time.

Most of my patients and those of my homeopathic colleagues, myself included, have avoided taking prescription drugs for decades. In my case, I have not taken a prescription drug of any kind since 1997 when I first became a homeopathic client. Severe fatigue, insomnia, and hypertension were the main conditions that plagued me. As a medical doctor, I knew that conventional treatment offered me only a lifetime of prescription drugs to treat the high blood pressure and there were no good pharmaceutical options for my other problems that didn't involve habit-forming drugs with many side effects.

I am forever grateful for what homeopathy has done for me and for my family. It is my humble privilege to share what I have learned with others and to offer hope to all who suffer with chronic disease that the art and science of homeopathy is available to help them too.

Homeopathic remedies are made in a special way in licensed homeopathic pharmacies by diluting and shaking, or succussing, a concentrated mother tincture of any natural substance. As the tincture is repeatedly diluted and shaken, the physical characteristics of the substance lessen as the energetic or healing properties are increased. In this way, substances such as snake venom or other poisons can be safely used to stimulate the Vital Force that knows innately how to restore a being to a state of health. The diluted substance is then poured onto milk sugar tablets, which act as a carrier for the energy released during the process of dilution and succussion. Thus, a remedy of 6c potency has been serially diluted in 100 drops of water six times and a remedy of 30c potency has been diluted 30 times. The mother tincture can be diluted an infinite number of times and the higher the dilution, the more potent the remedy and the greater its innate healing power.

In order to determine what remedy is needed by a sick person, a trained homeopath takes the case by listening carefully to the patient's life story. This includes information about the mental, emotional, and physical circumstances that surrounded the onset of the illness. By matching those symptoms and conditions with the information codified in all the provings of over 5,000 remedies tested on human volunteers, a homeopath chooses the "similimum": the one remedy that will stimulate the Vital Force to restore the patient to health.

In this way, homeopathic remedies can be used to treat whatever sickness afflicts a person by getting to the underlying cause of the disease, rather than merely suppressing, or covering up, symptoms like pharmaceutical drugs do. Every complaint that afflicts humanity from depression and anxiety to high blood pressure and chronic fatigue syndrome can be treated with the proper homeopathic remedy. There are remedies that work for everything from colds and flu to manic-depressive illness. The remedies are safe, effective, and ridiculously cheap! You can buy 85 doses of a single 30c potency in the health food store for under $10. Higher potency remedies can be ordered from homeopathic pharmacies and the cost varies but they are almost always less expensive than pharmaceutical drugs.

However, it requires a certain skill to properly choose the correct remedy to restore a person to health. Taking the incorrect remedy won't do any harm; it just won't have any effect on the illness. The only possible side effect of taking homeopathic remedies can occur if too much of the correct remedy is taken too frequently. This is known as a homeopathic aggravation. It is usually self-limiting and can be effectively antidoted to stop the effect of the remedy with simple things like coffee or strong mint. (More about that later in the book.)

To illustrate how homeopathic remedies work, consider an all-too-common ailment most people experience at least once in their lives: food poisoning. When a tainted food is eaten, there is an energy that is consumed with the substance. Hahnemann called this "a morbific influence inimical to life." This morbific influence disrupts the Vital Force, which responds by trying to fight back by causing vomiting and diarrhea. Stomach cramps and fever alternating with chills are also part of the symptom picture. These are the very same symptoms that showed up in volunteers who took a 3c potency of **ARSENICUM ALBUM** in the original proving. The symptoms of food poisoning are the same symptoms that show up when someone is poisoned with arsenic. By diluting the arsenic 30 times, the homeopathic pharmacist makes a remedy that can be safely given to the ailing person to help the Vital Force fend off the effects of the morbific influence. As a rule of thumb, the more severe the symptoms, the more often the remedy is given. In the initial stages, the remedy can be given every 15 minutes and slowly tapered off as the symptoms subside.

In this book, it is my intention to help you become your own homeopath in acute situations. Of course, this book is not meant to replace your own doctor or homeopath who may be treating you for chronic conditions. Rather, it is specifically designed to help you treat yourself or your family members for common ailments that are usually short lived or self-limiting. Although homeopathy can be used to treat other more serious conditions as discussed previously, that is not the focus of this book.

So, let the learning begin. I promise you that it will not only be interesting, but that you will be able to start applying your new knowledge right away.

Chapter 1

How to Take a Remedy

Homeopathic remedies are essentially little balls of energy that get released when they dissolve under the tongue. They are specially made in a homeopathic pharmacy licensed by the United States Homeopathic Pharmacopoeia.

To take the remedy, pour one or two pellets into the cap of the bottle and pop them under your tongue. It's best not to handle the pellets directly. Although the instructions on the bottle may recommend taking five to 10 pellets, it's not necessary to take more than one at a time—the number of pellets doesn't matter, but the frequency does. Remember, the remedy is just a carrier for the energy and it doesn't matter if you take one or 10 pellets, it counts as only one dose. Taking 10 pellets doesn't make the remedy work any faster—it just increases your sugar intake. However, taking one pellet 10 separate times a day means you would be getting 10 separate doses. This is rarely indicated except in acute cases where the symptoms are very severe and frequent dosing is required.

It is best to take the remedy separate from food or drink to allow the healing energy of the remedy to be released without interference from other substances. However, if it's a choice between waiting 20 minutes and skipping the remedy, take the remedy. Your Vital Force will figure it out.

Because the remedies work energetically to stimulate your Vital Force, there are a few things that can hinder or slow down their healing effects. There is some controversy among homeopathic practitioners about the effects of coffee. Some homeopaths are quite strict and forbid their clients from ever using coffee while they are undergoing homeopathic treatment. In my practice, I have seen a wide variety of reactions to coffee. Some of my clients can drink it without it interfering with the remedy whereas others cannot.

I remember years ago, I had a client who misunderstood my instructions and she took the remedy too many times in the course of a day. She called me in a bit of a panic as her symptoms had gotten considerably worse because she had effectively done a "proving" on herself by taking it too often. I had her breathe in the fumes from a bag of coffee beans and within 15 minutes the reaction stopped. This is a rare occurrence and can be avoided by taking the remedy as directed. (For more information on how a remedy is proven, see my first book VITALITY! How to Get It & Keep It: A Homeopath's Guide to Vibrant Health Without Drugs, available at Amazon and on Kindle.)

Nevertheless, while you are taking a course of homeopathic treatment, initially it is best to avoid or limit your intake of coffee for the remedy to work most effectively. Once you experience the clear benefit of taking the remedy for a while, you can add coffee back to your diet and see how you feel. If your symptoms return, then you will know that coffee is interfering with your remedy. Then you can choose which you prefer: your coffee or your symptoms. Strong mint can also interfere with some remedies so it's best to avoid taking breath mints or eating a lot of fresh mint during the course of treatment. Mint toothpaste is generally okay but I recommend staying away from those that have higher concentrations of mint, such as Tom's of Maine spearmint or peppermint. You can resume using them after you have finished the course of treatment. Other toothpaste brands like Colgate or Crest don't contain enough mint generally to interfere with the remedy. Choosing another flavored toothpaste such as anise, cinnamon, or lemon is another option also.

How often should you take the remedy in an acute situation? The general rule of thumb is, the more severe the symptoms are, the more frequently you need to take the remedy. For example, not too long ago, I got a nasty case of food poisoning from a sandwich in the Denver airport on the way to a skiing vacation in Utah. Within 30 minutes of eating, I began to feel light headed. Because I have been using homeopathic remedies for more than 25 years, my system is very sensitive to any morbific influence inimical to life that happened to be traveling with my lunch that day. (For most people who have not used homeopathy regularly, it often takes 12 to 36 hours for the body to show signs of illness after eating tainted food.)

By the time we landed in Salt Lake City, I had a full-blown case of all the usual symptoms: stomach cramps, cold sweats alternately with hot flashes, severe nausea, and, unfortunately, vomiting. (Thank God for air-sickness bags.) Fortunately, I never travel without **ARSENICUM ALBUM** in my homeopathic travel kit. I started taking the remedy every 15 minutes. As often happens, the vomiting increased as my Vital Force fought back against the energy of the bacteria in the food. This often happens as the body tries to purge itself. Of course, my travel companion had to pull the car over a few times on the way to the resort as the purging continued. Once the vomiting subsided, I took the remedy about every hour. Once we reached the resort, I slept for about an hour and when I woke up, I was completely well. The next morning I ate a big breakfast and skied the next 3 days without any residual effects. I continued the remedy daily for about 5 days to prevent a relapse.

The point of this tale of travel misery is this: take the remedy frequently at the beginning when the symptoms are most severe. As you feel improvement, cut back on the remedy to every few hours. Caveat: Don't stop the remedy once your symptoms go away. Instead, continue to take a dose once or twice a day until you are completely free of symptoms for about 3 days. Otherwise, your symptoms may return because a little bit of that morbific influence is still swirling around in your energy field.

Frequently Asked Questions about Taking Homeopathic Remedies

How do I know which potency to take?
The most common potencies available over the counter are 6c and 30c. In acute situations, choose the 30c. The 6c is usually given as a daily dose for chronic conditions at the beginning of a course of treatment. I also recommend the 6c potency in infants and small children; if a well-chosen remedy doesn't seem to be working, you can always switch to the 30c.

Do I need to stop my regular medications from my doctor?
No. Just take the remedies after you take your regular medications, if any. This is because the medications may slow the effect of the remedy. However, because the remedy works energetically, not biochemically, it won't interfere with any pharmaceutical drugs you may be taking. It's best to have at least an hour in between taking your meds and the remedy but do the best you can. You should

4

never stop any pharmaceutical meds abruptly without the advice of your health care practitioner.

What if I take the "wrong" remedy?
Homeopathic remedies work by resonating with the unseen energy of your Vital Force unlike conventional pharmaceuticals or herbs that work biochemically. For the remedy to work, it must match your symptoms closely enough to create this resonance. If the wrong remedy is chosen, the symptoms will persist; in other words, nothing will happen. This is why people often tell me, "Well, I tried homeopathy but it didn't work."

Can I take too much of a remedy?
Yes. As discussed, it's not the number of pellets that you take, it's the frequency of the dosing that can aggravate your symptoms. If the reaction is intolerable, you can antidote it with coffee or strong mint. In cases where a "constitutional" remedy is taken daily for a chronic condition, taking the remedy every other day or even every 3 days is usually sufficient to lessen the symptoms. This usually requires consultation with a professional homeopath and is beyond the scope of this book. But, for acute cases like food poisoning, fever, or ear infections, it will be clear when the remedy is wearing off and another dose is required. As you get used to using homeopathic remedies regularly, you will get a sense of when you need to take a dose and when you need to back off.

Where do I get these remedies?
If you have shopped in the homeopathy section of your local health food store, you have probably seen the display of "little blue tubes" made by Boiron. These are single-remedy vials made in either 6c or 30c potency. You can also order most remedies online from a homeopathic pharmacy. Certain remedies, called nosodes or

sarcodes, require a prescription from a homeopathic provider. All the remedies covered in this book are available over the counter with a few exceptions. The exceptions are available for order online. (For a list of homeopathic pharmacies, see Resources.)

Why should I pour the remedy into the cap rather than touching it with my fingers?

Because the remedies work energetically, there may be something on your fingers that could contaminate the remedy.

What's the difference between a single remedy and a combination remedy?

Single remedies are made from only one substance. For example, **ARNICA MONTANA** is a remedy for trauma made from a plant called leopard's bane. There are remedies that contain **ARNICA** in combination with other remedies, usually of the 6x potency. A remedy of 6x potency means that the original mother tincture has been diluted in 10 drops of water six times. The X (10) potencies are less potent than the C (100) potencies because they are less diluted.

In general, I recommend the single-dose remedies specific for your set of circumstances. However, there are some combination remedies available over the counter. In circumstances when you are too sick to think through which remedy to choose, taking a combination remedy for short-term relief may be your best approach. However, I consider this more of a shotgun rather than a laser approach. Taking the one remedy that best suits your symptoms is preferable and often works more quickly and deeply.

How do I get my remedies safely through airport security?

X-rays will cancel the effectiveness of homeopathic remedies so they cannot go through the X-ray machine at the airport. They can go through the metal detector. When I travel, I carry my remedies in a bag used for photographic film. I empty the tubes out into the plastic buckets provided for keys and change and give them to the TSA agent and ask for them to be hand checked. I then put the empty film bag, which is lead lined, through the X-ray machine.

I don't recommend packing your remedies in your checked luggage, even in a lead-lined bag. All baggage is X-rayed before it's placed on the plane. When the agent sees a dark image on the screen where the X-ray doesn't penetrate, they must open your suitcase and do a hand check. My concern is that when they open the lead bag and see the remedies, they may not understand what they are and put all the remedies through the X-ray machine.

One of my patients had this experience and when she got to her destination, she found none of her remedies worked while she was on her trip. She then had to buy all new remedies when she returned home.

I often give my patients a signed note on a prescription pad asking for the remedies to be hand checked. Ask your doctor to write one for you if they are willing to do so.

The ease of traveling internationally with remedies depends on the country. A few years ago, I was returning from Europe and I explained to the screening agent in a small airport in the Balkans that my remedies could not be X-rayed. He absolutely insisted that everything had to go through the X-ray machine. So, I put the remedies in their lead-lined pouch and he happily put the entire bag through the machine. No harm, no foul and my remedies were fine.

One of the advantages of traveling internationally is that homeopathic remedies are more readily available in most pharmacies, especially in Europe, India, and the UK. However, if you are traveling to remote places or locations where they don't have a health food store, carrying your own remedies is a blessing.

Can I take more than one remedy at a time?

Yes. Oftentimes, an additional remedy will be needed during a bout of illness. You can take them together, taking the remedy of the higher potency first. For example, if you were taking **FERRUM PHOSPHORICUM 30c and BELLADONNA 200c** for a *cold with a high fever*, you would put the 200c pellet in your mouth first, followed by the 30c pellet. It's not necessary to wait for the first pellet to dissolve before taking the second one. Remember, you only need to take one pellet, not 5 to 10, of each remedy. Otherwise, you would be taking a sizeable mouthful of sugar during the course of treatment.

Now that you understand how to take a remedy properly, how do you decide what remedy to take when you are sick? The simplest answer is to match your symptoms with the symptoms produced in healthy people during the original proving of the substance. For it is only by taking the remedy that is the most similar to your symptoms that your symptoms will be relieved.

If you have ever stood in front of the display of homeopathic remedies at the natural foods store, you know it can be a bit confusing as there are several remedies indicated for each condition. It is my intention to help you sort out this confusion by giving you a more detailed understanding of each of the most common remedies used for the most common conditions.

Chapter 2
Acute, Treatable Conditions
———— ɛɷʒ ————

ABDOMINAL BLOATING
———— ɛɷʒ ————

There can be many reasons for abdominal bloating, oftentimes with excessive intestinal gas buildup. The most common reason is that you're not tolerating something you're eating. Dairy products, especially in older people, wheat gluten, and of course beans are common culprits. Keeping a simple food diary or just paying close attention to what you've eaten in the prior 2 to 3 days can help you sort out the mystery. In the meantime, if you're experiencing **bloating and gas with or without abdominal cramping**, the first remedy to choose is **LYCOPODIUM CLAVATUM**.

It has a peculiar signature in that the complaints that call for this remedy are usually **worse between 4 pm and 8 pm**. So, if you notice that your digestion is usually most upset around dinnertime, give **LYCOPODIUM** a try. I've seen it work very quickly and it's healthier than taking simethicone, which is the active ingredient in most over-the-counter drugs for gas.

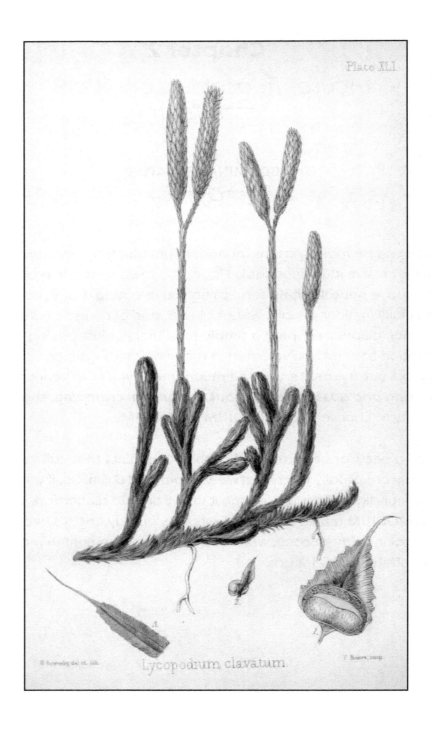

Plate XLI

Lycopodium clavatum.

ABDOMINAL CRAMPING

At times, flatulence, or gas, can be so severe that it causes severe *cramping* in the belly. Although the *Materia Medica* lists over 160 remedies for cramping pain due to gas, **LYCOPODIUM** and **NUX VOMICA** are the most readily available over the counter or in your emergency kit. Both of these remedies have cramps in their symptom picture, which means when they were tested in humans in their original provings, a large number of the provers developed cramping abdominal pain.

What distinguishes the two remedies, however, is the personality type. People who consistently need **LYCOPODIUM** as a constitutional remedy tend to have a *mild disposition*, somewhat indecisive at times and predisposed to worry about the details.

NUX VOMICA, on the other hand, tends to suit hard-driving business people who work too hard and crave alcohol to soothe their stress.

CARBO VEGETABILIS is another remedy indicated for marked *abdominal distention from gas* that is so painful it forces you to bend over. Unlike the other two remedies, there is usually marked *weakness, almost lifelessness, with some shortness of breath* in people who need **CARBO VEG**. It's commonly used for older, debilitated people after they have suffered a long illness.

If you're not sure which remedy to try first, I would suggest taking the **NUX VOMICA** if *cramping* is the predominant symptom. If *flatulence* is the main problem, go with the **LYCOPODIUM** first. In either case, if one doesn't bring relief after a few doses, try the opposite remedy. There's no harm in trying more than one remedy; just give it a bit of time before you switch. A rough rule of thumb I often use is to repeat the remedy every 30 minutes. If there's no change at all in your symptoms after three or four doses, try a different remedy.

ALLERGIES

No matter what climate you live in, seasonal allergies are a common problem for which homeopathy offers help in many forms. Choosing the right remedy requires paying close attention to the type of symptoms you're having. Do your eyes itch or do they burn? Do you sneeze or not? Does your throat tickle and then cause you to cough? Do you have sinus pressure or pain? Do you swell up like a puffer fish when you eat something your body doesn't like? Each of these symptom pictures is a guide to a different remedy.

Although there are close to 200 remedies listed for seasonal allergies, we focus here on those remedies most readily available in your local natural foods store. People who have suffered with allergies every year for most of their life benefit most from constitutional, ongoing treatment with a professional homeopath. However, there are several remedies that can bring relief in acute situations.

If you have ever chopped an onion with tears streaming down your face, then you know what it's like to need **ALLIUM CEPA**. This remedy, which is made from red onion, can bring almost instant relief for **red, burning eyes with lots of tears** brought on by environmental allergies. Although the eyes can feel itchy, the hallmark symptom of **ALLIUM CEPA** is a sensation of *burning irritation*. **EUPHRASIA OFFICINALIS** is the go-to remedy when there is marked *itching of the eyes* with a lot of *sneezing*. One of my patients who needed **EUPHRASIA** described wanting to "take my eyeballs out, give them a good scratching, and put them back in!" This is a perfect description of someone needing **EUPHRASIA**, especially when they can't stop sneezing.

When something in the air causes the whites of the eyes to become red *(conjunctivitis)* and the edges of the eyelids to swell, **HISTAMINUM** is the preferred remedy. This is especially true if there is also a feeling of the *ears being plugged up or blocked*.

When *postnasal drip with thick yellow discharge* is the symptom picture, choose **HYDRASTIS CANADENSIS**. There is usually a loose rattling *cough* and *irritability*, all made *worse by ingesting alcohol*.

NATRUM MURIATICUM is the remedy of choice in cases where *hay fever* brings on fits of *coughing so bad that the eyes overflow with tears*. *Runny nose* and severe *sensitivity to light* are also clues that **NAT MUR** is the remedy to take.

One of the most alarming, uncomfortable, and potentially life-threatening allergic reactions is hives, also called *urticaria. Urticaria* are red, raised, and often itchy lesions that can appear anywhere on the body. The most dangerous kind of hives are those that appear in the throat or the respiratory tract as they can interfere with breathing. In severe cases such as this, there are several remedies to take on the way to the hospital.

The first remedy to take is **APIS** to help counteract the intense *swelling* that may be obstructing the breathing passageway, or trachea. Take the 30c *every 15 minutes* along with **RHUS TOXICODENDRON. RHUS TOX**, made from poison oak, is not only helpful for hives but it is the first remedy to think of in cases of *shingles*. The other remedy often used for hives is **URTICARIA URENS**, or poison nettle. This remedy is helpful for people who suffer from seasonal allergies that manifest as *hives with intense itching of the skin*. **RHUS TOX** tends to be a deeper acting remedy; it is one of our most reliable remedies in the treatment of *arthritis*. (See the section on bone and joint pain.) When hives manifest and the joints are stiff, especially on waking in the morning, take the **RHUS TOX** first.

In a life-threatening situation, such as hives in the trachea or throat there is often **panic** or **anxiety** as breathing becomes affected. In addition to the **APIS** and **RHUS TOX, ACONITUM NAPELLUS** is very helpful for anxiety during or after a near-death experience. You can take it every 15 minutes with the other two remedies and taper off as the panic subsides. These remedies can be given on the way to the hospital and will not interfere with any other medical treatment. Determining and treating the underlying cause of hives requires professional homeopathic guidance. These remedy recommendations are intended only as acute support during an emergency as you seek professional help.

ANXIETY

Anxiety and panic attacks can be some of the most rewarding conditions to treat homeopathically because the remedies can provide relief without psychiatric drugs, which can often be habit forming and have unwanted side effects. As we discussed briefly in the section on allergies, **ACONITUM NAPELLUS** is one of the most potent remedies for *anxiety* and *panic attacks*. It's the remedy that probably every soldier who sees combat needs at some point. The hallmark symptoms of **ACONITE** are *fear of dying, panic attacks,* and *extreme anxiety* that come on after *shock of any kind* (physical, mental, or emotional). It is made from monkshood, which was commonly used (in nondiluted, nonhomeopathic form) as a poison in the Middle Ages. When **ACONITE** is needed, *numbness, tingling*, and *coldness* can appear in any part of the body but usually the extremities. A curious symptom indicating the need for **ACONITE** is *hot hands and cold feet*.

As we will see in the section on colds, **ACONITE** is also a great remedy for *upper respiratory tract infections*. Another hallmark symptom of **ACONITE** is *suddenness of onset*. A *cold or flu, usually with headache*, that comes on *suddenly after exposure to cold wind* calls for **ACONITE**.

This remedy can also be used to treat *chronic anxiety* of long-term duration. It is one of a constellation of remedies used to treat *posttraumatic stress disorder (PTSD)*. Of course, treating such serious conditions as this long term requires professional care. Oftentimes, giving **ACONITE** during a crisis where there is *shock, anxiety, and panic* will prevent long-term persistence of these symptoms because the remedy supports the Vital Force and removes the energetic imprint that causes long-term problems.

Two other remedies for anxiety that are readily available over the counter are **ARGENTUM NITRICUM** and **GELSEMIUM SEMPERVIRENS**. These remedies have many symptoms in common such as *fear of heights, stage fright, and ailments from anticipation*. People needing either of these remedies get nervous before taking a trip or before a big event. So, if you're feeling anxious before you have to give a speech in front of your boss and all your coworkers, how do you know which remedy to choose?

There are a few things that distinguish these two remedies. People who need **ARGENTUM NITRICUM** tend to *be hot, agitated, and talkative*. When **GELSEMIUM** is indicated, the mental picture is more one of *exhaustion, low spirits, and wanting to be quiet and left alone*. **GELSEMIUM** people tend to be *chilly* except when they are sick with flu and running a fever. **ARGENTUM NITRICUM** is the remedy most often used for *fear of flying*, although I have seen **GELSEMIUM** help nervous fliers when that was the only remedy available.

There's also a peculiar feature about **ARGENTUM NITRICUM** that is distinctive for this remedy. I often use this question when trying to decide if this is the correct remedy: "How do you feel when you stand on the sidewalk and look up at a tall building or skyscraper?" For folks needing **ARGENTUM NITRICUM**, the answer is something along the line of, "It makes me very nervous," or "I feel like the building is going to fall down on me." That's very distinctive only for **ARGENTUM NITRICUM**.

GELSEMIUM SEMPERVIRENS, on the other hand, is often a remedy indicated for the *flu*; its symptom picture includes *body aches, chills, and headache*. Often when **GELSEMIUM** is indicated, *flulike symptoms* may accompany the *anxiety* and then pass as soon as the anxiety-triggering situation has passed.

When in doubt about which remedy is the right one, there is no harm in trying either one based on your best approximation of your symptoms with the symptom picture of the remedy. If there's absolutely no response after three or four doses, switch to the other remedy. However, these remedies are similar enough that there may be relief even if the remedy isn't exactly a bull's-eye choice.

IGNATIA AMARA is another remedy often indicated for *nervousness and hysterical reactions*. In my practice, the most common reason I recommend **IGNATIA** is for *acute grief*. When a loved one dies, especially if the death is unexpected, the Vital Force suffers a shock. For some people, this manifests as *uncontrolled crying, anxiety, and a feeling of just not being able to process what has happened*. I call this remedy the "funeral Valium." **IGNATIA** works energetically to support the Vital Force during the grieving process without the suppressive, numbing effect of tranquilizers. I tell my clients that it helps to "take the edge off" the acute grief so they can move through the experience of loss and still be present. Antianxiety drugs like Valium or Xanax may temporarily blunt the emotional intensity but they can also interfere with mental clarity and memory. It is healthier to experience a situation, no matter how painful, fully conscious and in control rather than in a drug-induced fog. Homeopathic **IGNATIA** offers the Vital Force emotional support without side effects or the dependency risk that can occur with pharmaceutical drugs.

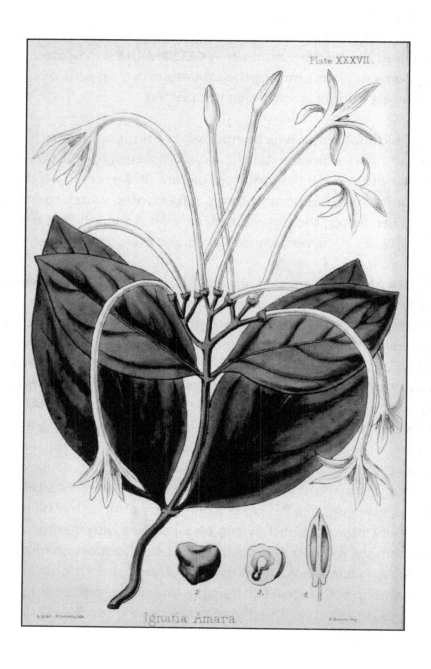

Plate XXXVII.

Ignatia Amara

have found this remedy also to be helpful for my patients on the anniversary of a loved one's death. Taking the 30c potency for a few days often helps when an event triggers painful memories that disturb your emotional equilibrium or disrupt your sleep.

Many other remedies have anxiety as part of their symptom pictures that were uncovered during the proving process. However, for acute situations, these three remedies are the most commonly indicated and readily available.

ASTHMA

Asthma is a condition of disordered breathing, oftentimes triggered by allergies to dust mites or animal dander. Its treatment is beyond the scope of this book. However, there are two remedies worth mentioning to use for someone having an acute asthma attack as you are heading to the hospital or doctor's office.

ACONITUM NAPELLUS, as we discussed in the section on anxiety, is helpful for the *panic* that often accompanies an acute, severe attack of asthma. The feeling of not being able to catch your breath often induces anxiety or a full-on panic attack. **ACONITE** given every 15 to 20 minutes at the height of the episode can have a calming effect and help ease respiratory distress.

CARBO VEGETABILIS is also another must-have remedy to keep close by if you or someone you love has asthma. **CARBO VEG** is a great remedy for *dyspnea, or shortness of breath*, where the breath is short, shallow, and difficult. Giving it every 15 to 20 minutes can often shorten or even abort an attack. Once the attac subsides, it's usually helpful to continue the remedies at least once day for a few days to prevent a relapse.

BEDWETTING OR BLADDER INCONTINENCE

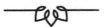

There are over 200 remedies listed in the *Materia Medica* for **incontinence, or loss of bladder control**, and obviously beyond the scope of this book. However, I mention it here because one of the remedies available in your local health food store, **CAUSTICUM**, is listed for **bedwetting and bladder incontinence**. As with the other 200-some remedies that help with this problem, the choice of remedy depends on the symptom picture elucidated in either clinical provings on sick people or in the original proving on healthy people.

In the case of **CAUSTICUM**, *leaking of urine* can occur *from the stress of coughing, sneezing, or laughing*. It's also indicated for *enuresis, or loss of urine, usually during the first few hours of sleep*. However, there are many other remedies that have these symptoms also. So, if you try **CAUSTICUM** for *bedwetting or stress incontinence* and it doesn't work, it doesn't mean that homeopath is not effective for incontinence. It just means you need a different remedy. An in-depth consultation with a professional homeopath can help.

BLADDER INFECTIONS

In the early days of practicing obstetrics and gynecology, I wrote hundreds of prescriptions for women suffering with chronic bladder infections. Oftentimes, these infections would be triggered by sexual intercourse, infrequent voiding (especially in teachers and nurses), or by dehydration from lack of adequate fluid intake. Becoming a homeopath was one of the best things I ever did for my patients who suffered from recurrent urinary tract infections (UTI) because I now have simple, inexpensive but effective remedies to offer them without the side effects of repeated courses of antibiotics.

One of my long-term clients came to see me for the first time 10 years ago because she had a history of bladder infections that recurred every few months. After so many repeated courses of antibiotics, the bacteria that constantly plagued her bladder were becoming resistant to the usual antibiotics. She was told that the next time she got an infection, she would need to go to the ER for intravenous antibiotics because the drugs normally prescribed for her by mouth were no longer working.

I took her case and determined a constitutional remedy for her based on her life's story and her medical history to boost her Vital Force. As often happens when people begin homeopathic treatment, her old UTI symptoms, which had been repeatedly suppressed with antibiotics, returned. By matching her particular symptoms with the symptom picture of the homeopathic remedy she needed, I added an acute remedy each time one of these old, suppressed infections would recur. Over several months, her recurrent bladder infections stopped completely because the remedies had succeeded in strengthening her Vital Force. Instead of taking an antibiotic that bypassed her own immune system, taking a homeopathic remedy enabled her own body's defenses to successfully eliminate the bacteria by sending more white blood cells to her bladder to eradicate the bacteria. Since starting homeopathic treatment and healing her Vital Force, she has not had one UTI in over 10 years and has not needed prescription medications of any kind for several ailments including fever, hives, and sinus infections.

As with all homeopathic treatment, the choice of remedy must be individualized. For example, let's consider the situations of two different women who both present with **painful, frequent urination and blood in the urine**. The first woman is 25 and just spent a week in Las Vegas on her honeymoon. The other woman is 76, living in a nursing home, and just got out of the hospital for hip replacement surgery. She had a urinary catheter in place during her surgery and for the first few days of her postoperative recovery. Although each woman presents with the same type of symptoms, the circumstances under which their Vital Force became deranged are completely different. Of course, they will each need a different remedy.

The younger woman needs a remedy called **CANTHARIS VESICATORIA**. Made from Spanish fly, this remedy is indicated when a bladder infection comes on from **very vigorous and frequent sexual activity**. There is also a **restlessness** that comes on when **CANTHARIS** is needed. It's difficult to get comfortable and there can be a **desire to pace or toss and turn in the bed**.

STAPHYSAGRIA is the remedy of choice when there is infection after **placement of a catheter**. **STAPHYSAGRIA** can also be used

22

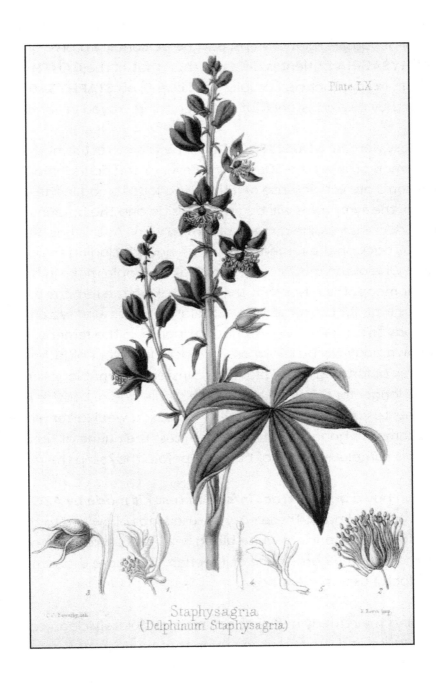

Plate LX.

Staphysagria
(Delphinum Staphysagria)

23

for a **UTI** that comes on ***after sex***, especially in women with a history of abusive relationships. But the personality profile of the **STAPHYSAGRIA** patient is different than that of the **CANTHARIS** patient. In my practice, I usually start clients on **STAPHYSAGRIA** first, unless they give a history that not everything stayed in Vegas!

For most women, **STAPHYSAGRIA** will be the correct remedy. I recommend taking the 30c potency every 1 or 2 hours initially if the symptoms are very intense or if there is a lot of blood in the urine. Usually the symptoms will begin to subside and the amount of blood decrease as the remedy begins to work. As this happens, you can cut back on the remedy to every 4 hours including through the night. One of the most common mistakes people make in treating UTIs homeopathically is that they stop taking the remedy too soon. It takes time for the remedy to stimulate the immune system and for the body to mount an appropriate response to the remedy. Because your own body will be killing off the bacteria in your bladder using an army of fortified white blood cells instead of antibiotics, it takes a little longer for the urine to become sterile again. I advise my patients to continue the remedy for at least a week after all their symptoms are gone. I then have them test their urine at home to be sure it is completely clear of bacteria before they stop the remedy.

You can buy a ***urinary tract infection test kit made by AZO*** online or at your pharmacy. These easy-to-use strips allow you to test your urine for the presence of white blood cells (leukocytes) and nitrite that indicate the persistence of infection. These are the same tests your doctor uses in the office.

Stopping the remedy before the urine is completely clean can lead to a relapse and the mistaken notion that homeopathic remedies don't work for treating bladder infections. I have seen it take as long as 3 weeks for the urine to clear in patients with a long history of multiple, recurrent UTIs. However, the good news is that, for most people, the symptoms go away long before the bacteria leaves the bladder completely. Taking the remedy until the urine test results are completely normal will usually prevent a repeat infection. Patience and perseverance are the keys to homeopathic treatment that reap the great reward of a life free of chronic antibiotic use.

Once you have successfully treated a bladder infection yourself without having to resort to antibiotics, you will be loath to take antibiotics again. Of course, the same proviso about when to see a doctor applies here as well. If you have tried a remedy or two and don't notice any change in your symptoms *or if you develop fever and/or low back pain*, you should seek professional assistance at once. Untreated bladder infections can spread to the kidneys in a serious infection called *pyelonephritis*.

While "pyelo" can be treated successfully with homeopathy, and I have done so many times, it is not something to be treated lightly and should always be treated by a professional with experience in treating serious illnesses. Oftentimes it requires more than one remedy over a longer period of time and the follow-up is critical to ensure that the infection is completely eradicated throughout the entire urinary tract. When it comes to treating kidney infections, as they say on television, "Don't try this at home!"

But a straightforward bladder infection with clear indications of which remedy to choose is a safe and relatively simple thing to treat if done correctly.

BONE AND JOINT PAIN

There are several types of bone pain and therefore many homeopathic remedies can be used to bring relief. For our purposes we will focus on two kinds of bone pain: *joint pain* and *pain associated with flu or other infections.* When trying to figure out which remedy to use for pain in the joints, the first question to answer is, "Is the pain worse or better with motion?" If you wake up in the morning with lower back or joint stiffness that is better once you get up and move around, the first remedy to consider is **RHUS TOXICODENDRON.** This deep-acting remedy has brought relief from *arthritis pain* to millions of people over the last 200 years in countries where homeopathy is widely practiced.

I have many clients who have had dramatic responses to this remedy. One of the most memorable is a woman named Pamela who was an obstetrics nurse for over 25 years. She had severe lower back pain that would radiate down her legs (*sciatica*). The pain was so bad when she woke up that she could not roll over in bed until she took 400 mg of ibuprofen. She did this daily for many years until she started homeopathic treatment. She started on **RHUS TOX** daily in the 6c potency with another remedy called **HYPERICUM** for the *sciatica*. Within 4 weeks she reported that she no longer required ibuprofen to get out of bed in the morning!

She has continued both these remedies in ever-increasing potency for the past 7 years and continues to be pain free most of the time. In fact, she recently took a month-long vacation hiking in the Alps, something she thought she would never be able to do. The hope is that eventually she will no longer require homeopathic remedies once her Vital Force completely recovers. Even so, for 7 years, she has not needed to take anti-inflammatory medications, which are not indicated for long-term use as they can have toxic effects on the liver and kidneys.

The usual symptom picture indicating **RHUS TOX** is the remedy of choice is that of a person who *awakens with stiffness in the joints* or other bones and feels a bit *better once they get up and get moving.* However, if they overexert themselves during the day, the pain will return. This remedy, which is made from poison oak, is also very helpful for *vesicular eruptions, or blisters*, brought on by *herpetic infections* such as *herpes* type 1 and type 2 and *shingles* due to *herpes zoster*. (See section on herpetic eruptions.)

Bone or joint pain that presents when the *slightest motion increases the pain*, calls for a different remedy called **BRYONIA ALBA.** The hallmark of **BRYONIA** is *motion aggravates.* This is true not only for bone or joint pain but for any condition that presents when the slightest movement makes the patient feel much worse. I have successfully used **BRYONIA** in my practice to treat cases of *acute appendicitis* (without surgery) and *pneumonia*. In both conditions, the patients could not move or breathe without experiencing excruciating pain.

One of the interesting things about these two remedies, **RHUS TOX** and **BRYONIA,** is that they illustrate the homeopathic principle of complements. I have treated patients over the years whose arthritis pain initially responded to **RHUS TOX**. After several months or sometimes years of relieving their pain with **RHUS TOX**, their symptom picture changed. The **RHUS TOX** no longer fit their symptoms and instead of feeling better when they moved, they felt worse. Stopping the **RHUS TOX** and changing to **BRYONIA** has often brought dramatic relief. This illustrates how important it is to pay attention to the details of each person's story. As their symptoms change, the remedy often needs to be changed as well.

However, these two remedies are not usually given at the same time. Either the pain is better with motion or worse with motion; in each case, the specific remedy is indicated but not both simultaneously unless there is an acute situation, like acute appendicitis, that gets superimposed over the chronic underlying condition. This is well beyond the scope of this book but I mention it only to emphasize that homeopathic remedies are tailored to each person individually and there is not just one remedy for one labeled condition or diagnosis.

EUPATORIUM PERFOLATIUM is one of my favorite remedies not only for the loveliness of its name but for the deep, almost instant relief it brings from pain so ***deep in the marrow, the bones feel as if they are about to break.*** This is a great remedy for severe bone pain that often accompanies ***flu*** or other ***deep infections*** such as ***dengue fever*** or ***Lyme disease***. One of my clients has been on a detoxification program to rid herself of chronic Lyme infection that she acquired years ago, after a tick bite. Periodically, as her body is purging the infection, she will develop severe bone pain. **EUPATORIUM PERFOLATIUM** has brought her almost instant relief when the pain was so debilitating she could barely get out of bed.

GELSEMIUM SEMPERVIRENS, the remedy we discussed for ***headache during the flu***, is another remedy that is very helpful in cases of flu when the body aches all over. Muscle aches in addition to pain in the bones and joints during the flu indicate the need for **GELSEMIUM.** The pain of **GELSEMIUM** that comes along with the flu is not as severe as the pain of **EUPATORIUM**; it's more of an ache than the feeling as if the bones are broken that comes with **EUPATORIUM.** When my clients complain of aching from the flu, I recommend they try **GELSEMIUM** first, especially if they have complained of *headache, slight chills, and they aren't thirsty.*

EUPATORIUM patients have more severe bone pain, primarily in the limbs, and less often complain of headache. Their fever is usually higher and alternates with severe chills. This was another remedy I found very helpful during the **swine flu** outbreak a few years ago. It's a remedy to consider in cases of severe bone pain due to more serious febrile illnesses like *Dengue fever, malaria, chronic Lyme disease, or swine flu.* Obviously, severe conditions such as these require professional care. But for travelers to exotic places where these conditions are endemic and health care may not always be readily available, having both these remedies in your emergency kit can make all the difference.

No discussion about bone and joint pain would be complete without mentioning *arthritis*. There are many forms of arthritis in conventional medicine: rheumatoid, psoriatic, and osteoarthritis, just to name a few. There are several hundred homeopathic remedies that can be used to treat various kinds of arthritis. The choice of the remedy depends not just on the diagnosis but also on the presentation of the whole symptom picture. Emotional and mental symptoms are just as important as the physical symptoms and are often the key to deciding which is the correct remedy.

As with any chronic condition, the correct remedy must be given and the potency adjusted over time. This requires professional care; although there are several over-the-counter remedies that can be used to treat arthritis when indicated, it is beyond the scope of this book. However, if you or someone you love suffers from arthritis pain, especially if you are considering taking conventional medications with serious known side effects, I would recommend a consultation with a well-trained homeopath in your area.

BROKEN BONES

Obviously, a fractured bone requires immediate professional attention. However, there are homeopathic remedies that are very helpful for **decreasing the time it takes a bone to heal** and **ensuring that the bone heals properly**. Remedies for trauma are discussed later in the book but while we're on the subject of bones, **SYMPHYTUM OFFICINALE** is a remedy worth special mention. Made from the comfrey plant, it is also known as "bone set" or "knit bone" because of its capacity to stimulate the Vital Force to direct the body's inherent capacity to build new bone. **SYMPHYTUM** is particularly well suited to fractures of the periosteum, which is the outer layer of bone. It is a great remedy for helping to heal **shin splints** or any bone **fracture, simple or compound**. I have used it in my practice to successfully treat full-blown **osteoporosis**.

My patient Betty's bone density returned to normal after many years of an abnormal DEXA scan result measuring 25% bone loss. After she suffered a broken wrist in 2012 and fractured the fibula bone in her leg in 2013, I had her continue to take **SYMPHYTUM** daily, even after the fractures healed, in ever-increasing potencies as part of her constitutional treatment (which included another remedy we'll meet in a moment called **CALCAREA CARBONICA**). In September 2014, Betty had a repeat DEXA scan that was completely normal. As in Betty's case, **SYMPHYTUM** is the first emedy to think of in women who have **recurrent fractures due to osteoporosis.**

CALCAREA CARBONICA, made from calcium carbonate, is also effective in treating **osteoporosis** and I have found the combination of both these remedies to be very effective for this common malady that afflicts many women around the time of menopause. However, each of these remedies needs to be given in increasing potency over time to effectively **reverse osteoporosis** and requires professional homeopathic consultation. There are other remedies that are indicated for osteoporosis and, like all homeopathic remedies, the choice of remedy is specific to each individual and should not be chosen only on the basis of a diagnostic label.

There is one very important thing to keep in mind when using **SYMPHYTUM** to facilitate bone healing. Because it is so effective at building bone, you should never take or give **SYMPHYTUM** until the fracture has been properly set and the proper bone placement verified by an X-ray film.

BREATHING DIFFICULTIES

Asthma, allergies, bronchitis, congestive heart failure, panic attacks, and pneumonia are just a few of the conditions that can cause respiratory distress. This book focuses on the remedies to take or give a loved one as you are heading to the ER.

As discussed in the section on asthma, there are two remedies available over the counter that are must-haves for anyone who suffers from breathing problems. **CARBO VEGETABILIS** is the first remedy to think of when you feel very *short of breath (dyspneic)* for whatever reason. It's especially well-suited for those who suffer with *congestive heart failure (CHF)*, in which the lungs fill up with fluid due to the weak pumping action of the heart. Of course, most people with *CHF* will be taking cardiac medications and this remedy is **NOT** meant to be a replacement for them. However, in a situation where there is *marked dyspnea*, especially *with exertion*, **CARBO VEG** can bring relief during the ride in the ambulance. Give or take the 30c potency every 20 minutes or so. In severe cases, the 200c potency can be given frequently and continued several times a day until the crisis passes.

CARBO VEG is also very helpful for people when they are in the process of *dying*. Often, breathing will be quite labored and **CARBO VEG** goes a long way in easing the *respiratory distress* that can sometimes come at the end of life.

BELLADONNA is another remedy indicated for *Cheyne-Stokes breathing* that often occurs during the dying process. This is a distinct breathing pattern in which there are periodic bouts of *apnea* followed by *deep* and *rapid respiration*. Giving **BELLADONNA** in the 30c or the 200c potency, depending on the severity, every 30 minutes or so can often bring relief from this breathing pattern that is not only difficult for the dying patient but is quite distressful for family members to watch.

Difficult respiration brought on by *panic attacks* often calls for **ACONITUM NAPELLUS**, the remedy for *shock*. Taking it or giving it every 30 minutes or so can bring considerable relief for someone in the middle of an *acute anxiety attack* brought on by any cause. The other tried-and-true method when someone is *hyperventilating from anxiety* is to have him or her breathe into a paper bag for a few minutes.

ANTIMONIUM TARTARICUM, as mentioned in the section on colds, is a remedy that can be almost miraculous in cases of *marked respiratory distress* during a severe *upper respiratory infection* when there is a large amount of mucus rattling around in the bronchial tubes and lungs. This remedy especially helps *children with a hoarse, croupy cough* who are *gasping for breath*. Be sure not to confuse **ANTIMONIUM TARTARICUM** with **ANTIMONIUM CRUDUM**. They sit side by side in the remedy display case at the store but they are two very different remedies. Give the 30c potency every 15 to 30 minutes on the way to seek medical attention to help ease breathing and relieve distress.

BRONCHITIS

The respiratory tract is divided into two portions: the upper and the lower. The upper respiratory tract includes the nasal cavity, the pharynx (upper throat and soft palate), and the larynx (voice box). The lower respiratory tract includes the trachea (windpipe), bronchial tubes, and the lungs.

The bronchi, or bronchioles, are the branching tubes that connect the trachea with the inner tissues of the lungs. Inflammation or infection of these tubes is called bronchitis. Acute bronchitis is caused by an infection or allergic reaction characterized by excessive production and accumulation of mucus. Chronic bronchitis is a long-standing inflammation of the bronchi often seen in smokers where the tissues are constantly irritated.

This section focuses on infections that spread from the upper respiratory tract to the bronchi. Treating infections of the lungs, called pneumonia, is beyond the scope of this book and requires professional care and advice.

Bronchitis typically develops from a cold that moves deeper into the chest. There are over 350 remedies that can be used for the treatment of bronchitis, but this discussion focuses on those that are readily available over the counter and are often the first remedies indicated when a bad cold becomes bronchitis (see also the section below on colds). The key to choosing the remedy is to accurately match your symptoms with the symptom picture characteristic of the remedy.

ACONITUM NAPELLUS is a remedy indicated for **upper respiratory infections** that **come on suddenly**, often after **exposure to a cold wind**. A **hot, throbbing headache** and a **hoarse, dry, croupy cough** that's **worse at night, especially after midnight,** are common symptoms that call for **ACONITE**. As with all remedies, taking **ACONITE** as soon as the symptoms manifest will often prevent the cold from progressing to **bronchitis**. Once the infection involves the bronchioles, the cough usually worsens, and there can be **difficult respiration with wheezing**. If the infection has been going on for a while, say a week or more, and has spread deeper in the chest, the 30c potency may not be strong enough. In cases like this, I recommend the 200c potency every 4 to 6 hours. Be sure to continue the remedy until all symptoms are gone for at least 3 days to prevent relapse. If taking the higher potency doesn't begin to bring relief, it's time to seek professional help.

ANTIMONIUM TARTARICUM, CARBO VEGETABILIS, DROSERA, DULCAMARA, FERRUM PHOSPHORICUM, and **HEPAR SULPHURIS CALCAREA** are all remedies that can be used in the treatment of bronchitis. Each of these remedies has a distinct constellation of symptoms that presents at the onset of a cold. Those same symptoms will be present in cases of **bronchitis** where the upper respiratory tract infection has moved farther into the chest often causing a **deep cough** and **chest pain on inspiration**. If you have been taking the 30c potency every 4 to 6 hours but the cold is not improving, there are two ways to proceed. If your symptoms still "match" the symptom picture of the remedy you chose, go up in the potency to the 200c and repeat it every 4 to 6 hours. If this doesn't bring relief within about 12 hours or your symptoms worsen, choose a different remedy. If your symptoms persist for more than a few days without any improvement or you develop a **fever,** it's time to seek professional help.

BRUISING

Any time there is trauma to the soft tissues of the body, in humans or in animals, bruising of the skin inevitably appears. The first and foremost remedy to take as soon as an injury occurs is **ARNICA MONTANA. ARNICA** was one of the remedies proven by Dr. Samuel Hahnemann himself. The idea for choosing this plant for a homeopathic proving came about after observing mountain goats eating this particular plant after falling while climbing on high, rocky cliffs. When given to healthy people in a proving, **ARNICA** brings on all the symptoms you would expect if you had just taken a header off your bicycle or been in a motor vehicle accident.

When taken immediately, **ARNICA** can prevent bruising almost completely. In my surgical practice, all my patients were given **ARNICA** before and after their procedures and their recovery was always faster than expected. By giving my surgical patients **ARNICA** in the immediate postoperative period, I was able to avoid the use of prophylactic antibiotics in almost every case. Boericke, one of our master homeopathic teachers, cites **ARNICA** for its ability to be a "prophylactic of pus infection." It is a common practice among plastic surgeons to give **ARNICA** before and after most procedures because it drastically *reduces the amount of bruising*, especially around the delicate tissues of the eyes.

One of my clients in Boulder, Moe Skaro, is a master healer and uses a unique technique called **PUSH** therapy that involves deep massage of the muscles and fascia. She also works on animals and she told me that she had been called to work on a horse that had been kicked in the shoulder by another horse. The wound had abscessed badly and the poor horse had been suffering from the wound for about 2 months despite several courses of antibiotics. Moe worked on the animal and advised the owner to give her horse **PYROGENIUM** in the 200c potency every 8 hours. Within 3 days all the pus was gone and the wound almost completely healed. She sent me the before and after photos and the improvement was striking. The combination of Moe's healing hands and the power of homeopathic **PYROGENIUM** saved the horse from going lame. However, I strongly suspect that if the horse had been given **ARNICA MONTANA** as soon as he was injured, the abscess could have been prevented.

PYROGENIUM is one of a special class of remedies called a **nosode**. It is actually made from rotten meat pus and has a powerful ability to clear up infection. I think of it as homeopathic antibiotics.

However, it is only available by prescription from a homeopathic pharmacy and requires special expertise to use it.

BURNS

CALENDULA OFFICINALIS is a must-have remedy in every family's medicine cabinet for the nearly miraculous relief it can bring for *burns.* From simple sunburn to a severe third-degree burn, **CALENDULA** is the first line of defense when the skin has been scalded or burned. It can be applied directly to the burn in either an ointment or a gel. I prefer the ointment as the gel usually contains alcohol, which can sting. For *second- or third-degree burns* involving deeper layers of the skin, I recommend taking the 30c pellet of **CALENDULA** under the tongue every 15 to 30 minutes in addition to applying the ointment often enough to keep the area moist.

CALENDULA is also very helpful for *cuts and scrapes*. When used with **ARNICA MONTANA,** it can *prevent wound infections* after surgeries, especially *after Cesarean section.* Be sure to continue taking **CALENDULA** at least once or twice a day until the skin has healed completely to minimize the amount of *scarring* and to *prevent infection*.

CALENDULA is also very helpful for *diaper rash.* You can apply it in ointment form but be sure the ointment *does not contain alcohol.* If that's not an option, dissolve one pellet of calendula 30c in water and apply it to your baby's skin and pat dry. You can apply it after every diaper change.

Although **CALENDULA** ointment is readily available in most natural food stores, the pellets are not. But you can order it online from a homeopathic pharmacy. The 2-dram bottle is usually sufficient as it contains about 85 doses. You may wish to order several vials to have on hand at home, in your car's first aid kit, and to store with your camping or travel gear. (See Resources for a list of homeopathic pharmacies.)

CANKER SORES AND COLD SORES

Canker sores, also known as aphthous ulcers, are open, painful sores that affect the mucous membranes *inside* the mouth. They can be white or yellow and are usually surrounded by red or inflamed tissue. They can occur on the gums or inside the lips or cheeks. They are most common in adolescents and young adults and they can recur several times a year. Stress, viral infections, or hormonal fluctuations associated with the menstrual cycle or with the onset of puberty can cause canker sores to erupt. Most of the time, they will heal within a week or two without treatment. But taking homeopathic **BORAX VENATA** 30c two to three times a day can bring pain relief and speed up the healing process. Unlike cold sores, canker sores are not contagious.

Cold sores are a different type of mouth sore caused by the herpes simplex virus. Unlike canker sores, cold sores usually erupt on the *outside* of the mouth around the lips and they tend to recur in the same place. Although there are over-the-counter and prescription drugs available to suppress a cold sore eruption, the homeopathic preparation of **RHUS TOXICODENDRON** is a better choice, in my opinion. When taken at the first tingling sensation that usually signals a cold sore, it can often prevent a full-blown eruption or limit its duration. It is also the first remedy to take at the onset of *shingles*, which is caused by another type of herpes virus called herpes zoster. **RHUS TOX** is especially helpful if the glands of the neck or under the chin are swollen during an outbreak. In my experience, taking **RHUS TOX** during recurrent outbreaks will often reduce their frequency or stop the recurrent pattern altogether.

COLDS

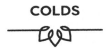

The commonly repeated bromide that "there is no cure for the common cold" is a myth. Homeopaths have been successfully treating colds for over 200 years. There are actually over 600 remedies listed in the *Materia Medica* for "coryza," which is essentially a cold. The first thing to consider is whether the symptoms came on slowly or suddenly. For a *cold that begins gradually*, usually with a sore throat, the first remedy to take is **FERRUM PHOSPHORICUM**. Take one pellet of the 30c potency under the tongue and repeat it every 4 hours. Sometimes taking the remedy early enough will stop the full-blown manifestation of a cold. Other times the symptoms can worsen to include a *severe sore throat, head congestion,* and *cough*. There are remedies that may be added for each of these phases of the cold, as discussed later. But the first remedy to take at the onset of a *cold that develops slowly* over a day or two is **FERRUM PHOSPHORICUM.** This is the same remedy to take *at the onset of any kind of inflammation* be it from a cold, a flu, or any type of infection. Of course, there are more specific remedies for various types of infections, which we cover later.

For **a cold that comes on suddenly**, especially after **exposure to a cold wind**, **ACONITUM NAPELLUS,** aka **ACONITE,** should be your first choice. I routinely carry a bottle of **ACONITE** in my ski bag. Oftentimes after riding a chair lift and skiing all day, by the evening, I'll have a cough or sore throat that comes on out of nowhere. Taking **ACONITE** right away gives complete relief without having to take cough syrup or cold medicine to sleep. With the proper homeopathic remedies, your Nyquil-swigging nights are over!

Sudden onset of a headache, sore throat, and a cough that's worse after midnight are all indications that **ACONITE** is needed. As we read earlier in the section on remedies for **anxiety,** an **ACONITE** cold can come on **after a shock** such as a car accident or a near-death experience.

If the cold moves into the chest, it can often cause a **cough**. There are several hundred remedies for cough depending on its quality. Is it a barking cough, a dry, hacky cough, or a wet cough? Is it worse lying down at night or worse in the morning? This is why there are several remedies listed for cough over the counter; each remedy covers a distinct constellation of symptoms. For our purposes, here, we review the cough remedies available over the counter and which remedy "matches" which set of symptoms. Most of the time, one of these remedies will do the trick.

ANTIMONIUM TARTARICUM is the remedy of choice when a **cough is wet, but nonproductive.** Often you can hear or feel mucus rattling around in your bronchial tubes but when you cough, no mucus comes up. This usually indicates that there is inflammation in the bronchial tubes of the lungs that is called **bronchitis.** A classic **ANTIMONIUM** cough is **worse in the morning.** Sometimes the cough can be so severe that it will make you **gasp for breath.** Other times, there will be **hoarseness of the voice from coughing.** An **ANTIMONIUM** cough doesn't usually have the **severe sore throat and hoarseness that indicates HEPAR SULPHURIS CALCAREA** is the needed remedy. If in doubt, you can take them both. There is often **drowsiness** when **ANTIMONIUM TARTARICUM** is indicated.

There is another similarly sounding remedy called **ANTIMONIUM CRUDUM,** commonly available in the same remedy display at the natural foods store. This form of **ANTIMONIUM** works primarily on the GI tract and is indicated for **indigestion with nausea.** Taking **ANTIMONIUM CRUDUM** when **ANTIMONIUM TARTARICUM** is needed won't relieve your cold symptoms.

DROSERA ROTUNDIFOLIA is indicated for a **deep, whooping cough** that is **worse lying down** and often **awakens you from sleep.** In the years before antibiotics, **DROSERA** was one of the remedies used to successfully treat **whooping cough,** also known as **pertussis.** If you suspect it's **whooping cough** in you or your child, take or give **DROSERA** every 30 minutes while on the way to see a doctor. Even if your doctor prescribes antibiotics, continue giving **DROSERA** until the cough is completely gone. Although the antibiotics will kill the pertussis bacteria, they do nothing to remove the energetic **morbific influence inimical to life** and the cure will be incomplete. This can lead to recurrent coughs or colds because the imbalance in the Vital Force that caused the predisposition to **whooping cough** in the first place has not been removed.

Although **whooping cough** can be and has been treated successfully without antibiotics, this requires the skill of an expert, highly trained homeopath and is well beyond the skill limits of the average person. While many purists would argue that you should never give antibiotics in lieu of a properly chosen homeopathic remedy, most laypeople don't have the requisite training or knowledge to manage such conditions. In my opinion, you should always err on the side of caution and seek medical help when you're not certain about the diagnosis or you don't see immediate results from taking a few doses of the remedy. You can always use homeopathic remedies to remove any side effects from drug treatment after the acute illness has passed with the help of a trained homeopath.

There is another remedy for a **whooping, rattling cough** that comes on after exposure to the **damp cold.** This remedy is called **DULCAMARA** and is indicated when the **cough is worse from physical exertion. DULCAMARA** is also very helpful for **hay fever with runny nose, worse from the nose becoming cold.** The hallmark of **DULCAMARA** is **aggravated from cold, wet weather.** The other indication that you need this remedy is **swollen glands, or adenitis.** So, if you develop a wet, rattling hoarse cough with marked swelling of the lymph nodes in the neck or under the chin, **DULCAMARA** is the remedy of choice. What distinguishes a **DULCAMARA cough** from a **DROSERA cough** is that the latter is always **worse lying down** and invariably requires **sleeping while elevated on pillows. DROSERA** doesn't have such a clear **aggravation from cold, damp weather** that **DULCAMARA does.**

HEPAR SULPHURIS CALCAREA is commonly indicated in the course of cold treatment. Its hallmark is **pain, especially in the throat.** When it's **painful to swallow and painful to cough, HEPAR** is the go-to remedy. The pain of **HEPAR** is described as a **splinter-like pain.** There is usually marked **hoarseness or complete loss of voice** when **HEPAR** is needed.

When there is purulence (that's the medical term for "pus") in the throat or the tonsils, especially with **pain in the ears**, think **HEPAR**. The other hallmark indication that **HEPAR** is needed is extreme **irritability or peevishness**. The **HEPAR** patient is overly *sensitive to everything* and often there is no pleasing them. It's best to give them the remedy and leave them be as fussing over them just irritates them more.

ARUM TRIPHYLLUM, made from the plant called Jack-in-the-pulpit, is fittingly a remedy for "clergyman's throat," which is an 18th century term for *laryngitis from overusing the voice*. Preachers at a tent revival, singers, circus ringmasters, or politicians on the stump can all benefit from **ARUM** when they lose their voices after hours of use or abuse.

SPONGIA TOSTA, made from toasted sea sponge, is a really helpful remedy when a *dry tickle in the throat brings on spasms of coughing*. It can also be used for *croupy cough* or for *"cardiac" cough* in patients suffering from congestive heart failure. The keynote symptom, however, is *severe dryness.* All the mucus membranes from the nose all the way down to the trachea feel "dry as a bone." Sometimes there can be a *fear of suffocation* during a severe bout of coughing when **SPONGIA** is needed.

COLIC

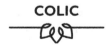

Is there anything more disheartening than the feeling of helplessness when trying to comfort a baby with colic? They cry almost nonstop and no amount of rocking or cuddling brings relief. Fortunately, generations of homeopaths have passed their wisdom on to us for the benefit of cranky babies and sleep-deprived parent everywhere.

The three main remedies for colic that are available over the counter are **CHAMOMILLA VULGARIS, COLOCYNTHIS,** and **LYCOPODIUM CLAVATUM.** The colicky baby who needs **CHAMOMILLA** will be ***extremely irritable.*** They are so intensely ***sensitive to pain*** that nothing brings them comfort. They ***want to be held*** all the time, they are ***hot and sweaty,*** and anything that brings ***warmth makes them worse. They are very sensitive to the slightest noise, especially music;*** singing a lullaby to them just makes them howl all the louder. Babies needing **CHAMOMILLA** will often have ***green, watery diarrhea*** that smells like ***rotten eggs.***

COLOCYNTHIS, made from bitter cucumber, is also a very helpful remedy for colic. Like **CHAMOMILLA** babies, the baby needing **COLOCYNTHIS** is often fussy but they give the impression that they are ***angry***. When a baby needs **COLOCYNTHIS,** they feel ***better when pressure is applied to their belly*** so it's not uncommon to see a colicky baby who needs this remedy trying to climb up your body when you hold them so they can press their belly against your shoulder.

One of the easiest ways to decide which of these two remedies to give is the ***hot water bottle test***. Try applying a warm compress or hot water bottle to your baby's belly. If they scream and throw it off the remedy to give is **CHAMOMILLA**. If it brings them comfort, give **COLOCYNTHIS**.

If neither of these remedies seems to fit your baby's symptom picture, the third remedy to consider is **LYCOPODIUM CLAVATUM.** Colicky babies needing this remedy will often have a very ***distended*** abdomen with lots of **rumbling noises** and plenty of **gas**. This usually occurs right **after eating.** One of the signature symptoms indicating **LYCOPODIUM** is the time of aggravation; the **LYCOPODIUM** baby *is worse between 4 and 8 pm*. Babies needing **CHAMOMILLA** are usually at their **worst during the night**. **COLOCYNTHIS** babies don't have as obvious a time of aggravation as babies needing the other two remedies often do.

With each of these remedies, when treating babies, I usually recommend starting with the 6c potency IN WATER. Simply put one or two pellets of the remedy in water and give it to your baby with an eyedropper or a teaspoon. I don't recommend giving the pellets to infants because of the rare risk of choking. You can give the remedy every few hours depending on the severity of the symptoms; the more they suffer, the more frequently they need the remedy.

If you give the 6c potency of the remedy and the relief seems to be short lived, that is, their symptoms keep coming back, give the 30c potency. Often the 30c once or twice a day should be enough. Of course, if your baby awakens in pain in the night, give another dose.

CRADLE CAP

Cradle cap is the common term for what dermatologists call *neonatal seborrheic dermatitis*. It's fairly common in infants and has a number of causes, ranging from antibiotics given to mom during pregnancy or to baby after birth, food allergies, and fungal infections. Hormones passed from the mother during pregnancy can cause the oil glands of the baby's skin to enlarge and secret an oily substance called sebum. This overproduction of sebum causes the skin to be irritated which usually manifests as a flaky, oily scalp but it can also affect the eyebrows, the eyelids, or skin around the ears.

In homeopathy, skin conditions are understood to be an indicator of a deeper imbalance in the Vital Force. Understanding the cause of this imbalance allows the proper choice of the correct homeopathic remedy to correct the underlying misalignment.

The reason I mention it here is that there is a homeopathic remedy called **CALCAREA CARBONICA** available over the counter that is often listed as a treatment for cradle cap. However, there are over 400 remedies listed in the *Materia Medica* of which **CALCAREA** is just one.

CALCAREA is indicated in cases when there is a lot of *sweating*, especially of the head. Children needing **CALCAREA** tend to be *less tolerant of cold weather*, are prone to *nightmares,* and often *crave eggs* or *eat dirt* (a condition known as pica). As mentioned elsewhere in the book, **CALCAREA** is a powerful remedy for other conditions such as *osteoporosis* and *menopausal hot flashes.*

Getting back to cradle cap, my advice would be to give it time before giving a remedy. In most cases, cradle cap will resolve on its own. However, if it persists or worsens over several months, that's an indication that the Vital Force is "asking for help." I would recommend a consultation with a homeopath who can assess the imbalance in the Vital Force and recommend the proper remedy to address the underlying cause.

DIARRHEA

First, I recommend *not* reading this section while you're eating! This is certainly not a pleasant topic to discuss and an even worse condition to have. But it is such a common malady that strikes most everyone at some time in their life and homeopathy has a wide variety of remedies that can bring relief.

As with any condition, there is both acute and chronic diarrhea. *Chronic, long-standing diarrhea* is an indication of a more serious internal imbalance and is beyond the scope of this book. Conditions such as *Crohn's disease* and *ulcerative colitis* can be treated successfully with homeopathy but require skill and training to understand the morbific influence inimical to life that is at the root cause of the disease, and it will be different for each individual. For our purposes, this book focuses on the two remedies that are readily available over the counter to treat **acute diarrhea**.

CHINA OFFICINALIS is made from the bark of the cinchona tree, which is native to South America. It was the source of quinine used to treat malaria for centuries before quinine was chemically synthesized. The homeopathic preparation has a wide variety of uses, especially for cases of *severe weakness after loss of bodily fluids.* But its availability over the counter is primarily intended to help bring relief from *traveler's diarrhea.*

Diarrhea brought on from *drinking bad water* or *eating unclean fruit*, especially if there is a feeling of *weakness* and lots of *abdominal gas and bloating,* indicates the need for **CHINA.** This remedy is discussed further in the section on **food poisoning** and in the **travel section** to distinguish it from another remedy that is also very helpful for travelers called **ARSENICUM ALBUM.**

There are also distinct mental and emotional symptoms that can guide you in choosing the right remedy. When **CHINA** is indicated, there is often a **restlessness of the mind**, especially **at night**. When people need **CHINA**, they will often lie awake because the mind is full of a **profusion of ideas** that keep sleep at bay. In the morning, they awaken **irritable and exhausted.**

PODOPHYLLUM PELTATUM is the other homeopathic remedy for diarrhea readily available in health and natural food stores. This remedy is indicated when there is **thin, green or yellow diarrhea that is painless and gushing.** The other distinguishing feature of **PODOPHYLLUM** is its **alternating characteristics.** Often there will be **diarrhea alternating with constipation** or **diarrhea alternating with headache** when **PODOPHYLLUM** is the needed remedy.

Use the 30c potency with either of these remedies and repeat it every few hours. As the symptoms begin to subside, cut back on the frequency but don't stop it entirely until all symptoms have been gone for at least 3 days.

EAR INFECTIONS

Otitis media is the clinical term for **infections of the middle ear**. Some children suffer with recurrent ear infections that require multiple courses of antibiotics, especially in the winter months.

Although the antibiotics, if prescribed correctly, will usually kill most of the bacteria causing pus and fluid to accumulate behind the eardrum, they don't do anything to address the underlying reason the infection developed in the first place.

Chronic, recurrent otitis media requires professional homeopathic consultation in order to avoid the repeated rounds of infections and multiple courses of antibiotics. However, if an ear infection is treated with the correct homeopathic remedy the first time, recurrent infections can often be prevented. This is because a properly chosen homeopathic remedy removes the morbific influence inimical to life that is the root cause of all infections, no matter where they manifest in the body.

Paying close attention to your child's symptoms and the circumstances that brought them on can help you to choose the correct remedy. In most cases, the 30c potency repeated every few hours gives relief from the pain and brings down the fever that often occurs. If you don't see any improvement after two or three doses, choose a different remedy and/or get professional help. As with any infection, if you decide to use antibiotics, it is still helpful to find the correct homeopathic remedy and give that also. The proper remedy will work to strengthen the Vital Force, remove the predisposition to infection, and help to prevent a recurrence.

With that understanding, there are several remedies available over the counter that can be used to successfully treat an ear infection. **BELLADONNA** is the first remedy to choose when there is *sudden onset of high fever* and *throbbing pain*. Children needing **BELLADONNA** are often very *sensitive to light and noise*. The *face is hot and flushed* and the *pupils of the eyes can be dilated.* **BELLADONNA** is a right-sided remedy; often the infection occurs in the right ear. However, don't hesitate to give this remedy for an infection of the left ear if the rest of the symptoms fit the **BELLADONNA** picture. **BELLADONNA** is a rather short-acting remedy, meaning that the conditions that call for it are often short-lived, lasting just a few days. Therefore, **BELLADONNA** is the first remedy to think of for *ear infections that come on suddenly with a high fever and usually last just a few days.*

In some cases, the fever will go away and the child starts to improve but the ear pain lingers. The red face is gone but now the child starts to *sweat*, especially *about the head*. This calls for a second remedy called **CALCAREA CARBONICA**, which is the "chronic" of **BELLADONNA**. Giving **CALCAREA** 30c two to three times a day will usually "finish" the infection. As with any infection, give the remedy at least once a day for 3 or 4 days after all symptoms are gone to prevent a relapse.

It is not uncommon to see ear pain or ear infections in *teething babies.* In these cases, the baby is *extremely irritable* and wants to be *rocked or carried all the time*. The ears are *very sensitive to* cold *wind or drafts*. There may be fever but it usually does not come on with the suddenness seen in **BELLADONNA**. This symptom picture calls for **CHAMOMILLA**, one of the remedies discussed in the *colic* section.

When **CHAMOMILLA** is needed, the *ears are very painful* and *sensitive to the slightest touch*. The other very distinct symptom that calls for **CHAMOMILLA** is that *one cheek is red while the other cheek is pale.* This helps to distinguish the case from **BELLADONNA** where both cheeks or the entire face are usually flushed and *bright red.*

There is one other remedy commonly indicated for ear infections that has this same peculiar symptom of *one red cheek and one pale cheek during fever*. That remedy is **PULSATILLA NIGRICANS**. The distinguishing feature of **PULSATILLA**, however, is *weeping.* Children needing **PULSATILLA** tend to have a milder disposition; they don't have the extreme irritability you see with **CHAMOMILLA** or the temper tantrums that can come with **BELLADONNA.** But they don't seem to be able to stop crying no matter what you try. They don't want to be left alone and can sit quietly in your lap for hours unlike the sick baby needing **CHAMOMILLA** who *demands to be carried* around the house because they *feel better moving about.*

The ear infections calling for **PULSATILLA** are *worse at night* and applying a warm compress to the ear does NOT bring relief. **PULSATILLA** is often the remedy needed for *mumps.* The other distinguishing characteristic of **PULSATILLA** is *thirstlessness.* The child needing **CHAMOMILLA** is often *thirsty for cold drinks*; the **BELLADONNA** baby wants something *sour* to drink like lemonade or lemon water.

Once again, to avoid any risk of choking, when giving homeopathic remedies to small children, it is best to put a pellet or two in water and give them a spoonful rather than giving them the pellet directly.

It may seem difficult trying to choose the right remedy, especially when your child is crying in pain. Patient observation and attention to detail go a long way in helping you to make the right choice. The more in tune you are with the changes you see in your child when they are sick, the more likely you will know what remedy to give. Of course, the more knowledge and experience you gain each time you use a homeopathic remedy, the more confident you will become.

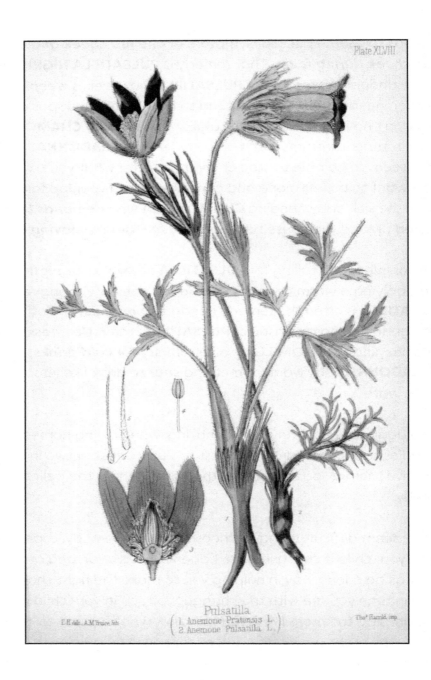

Plate XLVIII

Pulsatilla
(1. Anemone Pratensis L.)
(2. Anemone Pulsatilla L.)

Remember, you can always reach out to a homeopath in your area if you need professional help.

The reward of seeing your child drift off to peaceful sleep and awaken much improved and fever free after you have given a remedy is well worth the time and effort invested to learn more about these miraculous little pellets.

EYE DISORDERS

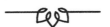

In the section on allergies, the common remedies available to treat burning or itching of the eyes associated with hay fever or food allergies were shared. This section covers a few other minor eye ailments for which remedies are available over the counter.

RUTA GRAVEOLENS is a wonderful remedy for *eye strain,* especially for those who spend hours each day reading from electronic screens. *Eyestrain from reading* for long periods of time, especially in dim light, calls for **RUTA.** In addition to the sensation of *fatigue*, the eyes can feel *as if they are on fire* when **RUTA** is needed. *Headache from eye strain* is another indication for **RUTA GRAVEOLENS.**

There are about 70 different remedies for *styes* but there is one remedy available over the counter that may help in a specific type of *stye*. **STAPHYSAGRIA** is the remedy to try for *styes* that never seem to "break open" but persist with a little hard nodule on the eyelid. Taking the 30c potency one or two times daily can help resolve a *stubborn, chronic stye*.

As in the section on allergies, **APIS MELLIFICA**, made from the honeybee, is a beautiful remedy for *swelling* of any kind. In severe allergic reactions, the eyelids can become so puffy it looks as if *little bags of water surround the eyes*. **APIS** is a godsend in these situations and can rapidly reduce swelling.

APIS can also be very helpful in cases of *conjunctivitis*, commonly known as pink eye. However, **APIS** is one of 236 remedies listed for *conjunctivitis* in the *Materia Medica*. It is the *swelling of the eyelids*, either upper, lower, or both, that indicates **APIS** when the conjunctiva, or white part of the eye, is *red and inflamed.*

BELLADONNA can also be used for conjunctivitis but the symptom picture is different. Like other conditions calling for this remedy, the eye inflammation *comes on suddenly* with *extreme redness*. Allen's *Primer of Materia Medica* describes the conjunctivitis of **BELLADONNA** as "so great that the eyelids are rolled outward." There can be *bleeding of the eyelids* and *severe sensitivity to light*. Obviously, in cases this severe, the remedy should be taken on the way to the eye doctor. Although pharmaceutical drugs may be prescribed, the remedy should be continued in order to treat the underlying predisposition that allowed the inflammation to start.

Conjunctivitis from trauma occurs when there is *bleeding in the small blood vessels* of the white portion of the eye. This bleeding can occur from a *foreign object* or even after a severe bout of *coughing*. In these cases when there is actual *hemorrhage of the small blood vessels,* the remedy indicated is **CALENDULA**. **CALENDULA** is also very helpful in cases of a *scratched cornea*.

Unfortunately, most health food stores only carry **CALENDULA** in ointment or gel forms that are not appropriate for use in the eye.

Most home emergency kits from a homeopathic pharmacy will contain **CALENDULA** in pellet form because of its ability to **prevent or stop bleeding.** Taking the 30c pellet orally several times a day will help speed the healing of the eye and clear the hemorrhage.

ARNICA MONTANA is the main remedy for trauma of all kinds, and **eye trauma** is no exception. **ARNICA** is especially helpful for **injury to the bones of the eye socket**. Giving **ARNICA** immediately and repeating it frequently after an injury can accelerate the healing process and prevent further complications.

FEAR OF FLYING

The *Materia Medica* lists 11 remedies for "fear of airplanes" and fortunately six of them are available over the counter. So, if you are afraid to fly, odds are that there is a remedy to help you. As with all homeopathic remedies, the key to choosing the correct one is based on how closely the totality of your symptoms match those of the remedy.

As we saw in the section on anxiety, **ACONITUM NAPELLUS,** or **ACONITE,** has a hallmark symptom of **fear of dying.** This is the remedy to use for fearful fliers who may have had some form of untreated **shock** in the past, who **startle easily,** and have developed a **phobia** around flying. When **ACONITE** is needed, there is usually a feeling of **restlessness**, **numbness, and tingling in the extremities** and a **desire to be out in the open air.**

Nervous travelers who need **ARGENTUM NITRICUM** suffer from *"ailments from anticipation."* They feel anxious days or even week before their trip and can often speak of nothing else. They often **fee hot**, their hands may **tremble,** and they **crave sweets.** They tend to **rush around** doing several things at once and are often **in a hurry**. (For more information about **ARGENTUM NITRICUM,** see the sectio on Anxiety.)

I was recently on a flight where a young woman sitting across the aisle clearly needed **ARSENICUM ALBUM.** She was very **pale** and had a death grip on the airsickness bag, most likely because she was **nauseated.** She had a severe case of the shakes despite wearing a heavy coat and a blanket. She demonstrated many of the hallmark symptoms of **ARSENICUM ALBUM: anxiety, chilliness, and nausea.** Once the plane landed, she was fine.

CALCAREA CARBONICA is not the first remedy we usually think of for nervous fliers but it's helpful in cases when the fear is more one of **claustrophobia.** People needing **CALCAREA** are often **exhauste from overwork** or **from taking on too much responsibility**. They tend to be **chilly** and can have the **cold sweats**. I have used this remedy successfully for **overwhelmed, working mothers** who must travel for their jobs and have developed anxiety every time they ge on a plane. **CALCAREA** helps to take the edge off. In these cases, they need **CALCAREA** for longer periods of time to help them restor their Vital Force that has often been depleted by **doing too much for too many people.**

LYCOPODIUM CLAVATUM is another less well-known remedy for **fear of flying**. The key symptoms that indicate **LYCOPODIUM** are lots of **intestinal gas** and a **time aggravation between 4 and 8 pn** One of my clients kept this in his travel kit because, invariably, every time he got on a plane, his belly would fill up with gas no matter what he ate. Fortunately for his fellow passengers, a few doses of **LYCOPODIUM** not only eased his *anxiety* but also worked better than any of the over-the-counter gas remedies he had previously tried.

The last fearful flier remedy available over the counter is **NATRUM MURIATICUM**, which is a common remedy for *headache* and is the remedy to think of when the *anxiety about flying* brings on a *headache that feels like a tight bandage* around the forehead and temples.

FEVER

Fever is a common sign of infection as it is one of the body's defense mechanisms against unwanted invaders. Rather than just suppressing a fever with medications like aspirin, acetaminophen (Tylenol), or ibuprofen (Advil, Motrin), homeopaths regard fever as a signal from the Vital Force "asking" for help in the form of a specific remedy. As expected, there are hundreds of remedies that have fever as part of their symptom picture. Here we discuss the remedies readily available over the counter and the most common conditions indicating their use.

There are two remedies to consider when there is *sudden onset of fever*: **ACONITE** and **BELLADONNA.** Although both have *suddenness* as part of their symptom picture, they have quite a few features that distinguish them from one another. In cases of fever indicating **ACONITE,** the *skin is dry* and there is usually some element of **anxiety** present. A **cold or flu with fever** that comes on suddenly after **exposure to cold**, often with **headache**, is the common symptom picture of **ACONITE**.

People needing **BELLADONNA** for **sudden onset of fever** often have a **flushed, red face** and tend to **perspire**. The fever can be quite high, often 102 degrees or higher, but once the remedy is given, it usually doesn't last long or tend to relapse or recur regularly as when some other remedies are indicated.

EUPATORIUM PERFOLIATUM is a powerful, often overlooked remedy for fever where the hallmark symptom is **severe bone pain**. This remedy proved to be a lifesaver for a child I treated who had the **swine flu** a number of years ago. **EUPATORIUM** brought almost instant relief from the bone pain and was one of six remedies she needed hourly for the better part of 2 days until the fever was finally gone. (Yes, her mother was a saint setting her alarm every hour to give her child a cocktail of remedies.) Obviously, this is not something to try yourself at home but in cases of **simple fever** when the **bones feel as if they are broken**, **EUPATORIUM** is a great pain reliever and fever reducer. It's also a common remedy for **DENGUE FEVER** and should be part of any serious traveler's first aid kit.

As we saw in the section on colds, **FERRUM PHOSPHORICUM** is the first remedy to think of at the **early onset of any type of inflammation.** In a cold that **begins slowly**, usually with a **sore throat** and a **low-grade fever, FERRUM PHOS** can often shorten the duration of the illness or prevent it from progressing to something worse. This slow onset of symptoms is one of the features that distinguishes **FERRUM PHOS** from **ACONITE or BELLADONNA** whose **symptoms tend to come on suddenly.**

GELSEMIUM is the go-to remedy for *fever and body aches due to flu.* One of the keynote symptoms of **GELSEMIUM** is *overwhelming weakness and fatigue.* People needing this remedy often don't feel like getting off the sofa, they feel *anxious,* and they want to be *left alone*. **GELSEMIUM** is one of the best remedies for *chronic fatigue syndrome* in people who have never been well since a bad bout of *flu*.

As we saw in the section on anxiety, people needing **GELSEMIUM** often suffer from *ailments from anticipation* (like **ARGENTUM NITRICUM**). They *dread going to the doctor* even when they are very ill. Giving **GELSEMIUM** when indicated for *flu* can restore the Vital Force and prevent long-term complications.

FLU

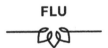

Although we have already discussed each of the following remedies, it bears mentioning them again in relation to their use for treating *gastrointestinal flu*. There are two kinds of flu: respiratory and gastrointestinal. *Respiratory flu* involves the upper respiratory tract, which includes the nasal cavity, the pharynx (upper throat and soft palate), and the larynx (voice box). *Gastrointestinal flu* manifests in the gut and its symptoms can include *nausea, vomiting,* and *diarrhea. Fever, headache, body aches,* and *fatigue* can occur in either type of flu.

FERRUM PHOSPHORICUM is the first remedy to take at the *early onset of any kind of inflammation* as occurs with colds and flu. **FERRUM PHOS** is indicated when the ***symptoms come on gradually,*** over a few days, and if there is fever it is usually of a low grade. As the flu progresses, it may be necessary to add another remedy as the symptoms change. It's a good idea to continue taking the **FERRUM PHOS** during the entire course of the illness as it helps prevent relapse.

As we just read in the discussion of **GELSEMIUM,** incomplete treatment of the flu can result in ***persistent weakness*** or even ***chronic fatigue***. **CHINA OFFICINALIS** is the primary remedy given when there is ***weakness*** or ***fatigue from loss of vital fluids***. This can occur in severe cases of flu where there has been ***prolonged vomiting and diarrhea***. Taking **CHINA** until the fatigue is gone restores the Vital Force and helps to prevent the long-term debility that can come from a severe bout of flu.

Severe bone pain during a bout of either respiratory or gastric flu calls for **EUPATORIUM PERFOLIATUM**. I have used this remedy with great success in several seemingly unrelated conditions where **pain deep in the bones** was the major symptom. In addition to helping a client manage the symptoms brought on by detoxing from Lyme disease, **EUPATORIUM** has also helped several of my patients who suffered with ***pain in the bones of the head*** where the usual headache remedies failed to work.

FOOD POISONING

In my experience, one of the most rewarding conditions to treat homeopathically is food poisoning. A properly chosen homeopathic remedy can shorten the duration of the illness, prevent dehydration, and save you a trip to the hospital for intravenous fluids and a 10-day course of antibiotics. I have had food poisoning on four separate occasions, usually while traveling, and **ARSENICUM ALBUM** has brought me through every time.

The symptoms that call for this remedy are *nausea, vomiting, diarrhea,* and *stomach cramps. Dizziness* or *light-headedness* can be one of the early symptoms. One of my clients suffers with a severe bout of *vertigo* when she needs **ARSENICUM ALBUM**. Take the 30c potency every 15 to 30 minutes at the first sign of trouble. As the remedy "does battle" with that morbific influence inimical to life, there will be a temporary increase in your symptoms as your body does its best to purge itself. As the *nausea, vomiting,* and *diarrhea* lessen in intensity, cut back on the frequency of the remedy to every hour, then every 2 to 4 hours until you begin to feel better. Take the remedy once or twice a day for a few days after all your symptoms are gone to prevent the fatigue that can often persist after a "boxing match" with tainted food.

CHINA OFFICINALIS is another remedy often indicated in cases of *food poisoning*. As discussed in the section on diarrhea, **CHINA** should be part of every traveler's first aid kit. It's the remedy to use when *watery diarrhea* is the main consequence from *eating or drinking contaminated food or water. Severe fatigue* persisting after a bout of *traveler's diarrhea* calls for **CHINA.**

In cases of *food poisoning* where *persistent vomiting* is the main symptom, **IPECACUANHA** is the remedy to consider. When this remedy is indicated, there is *no relief after vomiting*. The more the person vomits, the greater is the urge to continue vomiting when **IPECACUANHA** is needed.

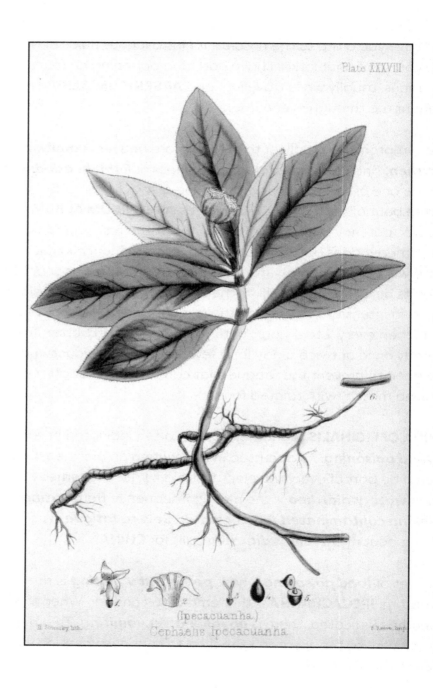

Plate XXXVIII

(Ipecacuanha.)
Cephaëlis Ipecacuanha

The homeopathic preparation of **IPECACUANHA** is made from the root of ipecac. The mother tincture is used to make syrup of ipecac, which is often given to induce vomiting after ingestion of some kinds of poison. It is not available over the counter but you can order it from a homeopathic pharmacy online. I recommend getting both the 30c and the 200c and carrying it in your travel kit.

GROWING PAINS

Have you ever wondered why one of your children has growing pains and the other does not? They have the same parents, they eat the same diet, and are both physically active, yet one child complains of pain in their legs, often waking them from sleep, and the other does not. Is it genetic? Is it something in their environment? Do they need vitamins?

Not necessarily. Most likely the child complaining of growing pains is in an energetic state that calls for **CALCAREA PHOSPHORICA.** Children needing this remedy will complain of *pain in both legs*, usually *at the end of the day,* and often *after they have been particularly active* playing sports or running around the playground. This is the child who will eat anything as long as it is wrapped in bacon or disguised as a hot dog because they *love smoked meats*. They can be a bit stubborn or hard to please and may sometimes throw a temper tantrum even years after the "terrible twos" have passed.

CALCAREA PHOSPORICA, made from calcium phosphate, has a particular affinity for the sutures or growth plates of the bones. Like the remedy **SYMPHYTUM OFFICINALE,** it can be used to treat people with *osteoporosis* or to help bones that are slow to *heal after a fracture* or in certain medical conditions where there is *delayed growth of the bones.* Giving the 30c pellet at bedtime or when your child complains of leg pain not only relieves pain but, over time, you may notice your child is less irritable and may even be open to trying other kinds of food.

HANGOVER

For many people, the holiday season involves lots of parties with lots of rich food and more alcohol than usual. **NUX VOMICA** is a lifesaver when you've imbibed too much of the "spirits" of the holiday. Taking the 30c potency before you go to bed and again when you wake up in the morning helps to detoxify your system and give your Vital Force some extra love. Alcohol tends to dehydrate the body so I recommend that you drink two glasses of water for every cocktail; 500 to 1,000 mg of vitamin C before bed with a large glass of water helps your liver to detoxify your system overnight.

NUX VOMICA is also a great remedy for *heartburn* or *gastric reflux,* especially after *eating rich or spicy food.* I have many clients over the years who have been able to stop using antacids or "the purple pill" after taking a course of **NUX VOMICA.** As a constitutional remedy, it's *especially well-suited to stressed out businessmen and women* who tend to overwork and then try to relax with a cocktail or two. I have seen this remedy help people decrease their **craving for alcohol** and rich, spicy foods as well.

HEADACHES

Before I did my homeopathic training, I would dread patients complaining of headaches. It was often difficult to determine the cause and invariably I would end up referring them to a neurologist who usually prescribed one or more drugs. The patients would report back to me that although their headaches occurred less often or were less intense, most all of them complained of side effects related to the medications they were taking. Inevitably, their headaches would recur and they would be prescribed more or different drugs in an attempt to get permanent relief.

However, once I became a homeopath, I understood that headache, like any other symptom the body produces, is just a cry for help from the Vital Force that has been weakened or depleted by something. When looked at from this broader perspective, it makes sense that headaches can appear as a result of grief, after a heart attack, during pregnancy or after childbirth, and certainly after someone has suffered a concussion, a head injury, or a whiplash from a motor vehicle accident.

Headaches can also be a side effect of certain medications or a sign that the neck or spine needs chiropractic adjustment.

This explains why there are more than 1,200 homeopathic remedies available to treat headaches; you can have 50 people complaining of headache and each of them may need a different remedy. The woman who has had daily headaches since the birth of her fourth child most certainly needs a different remedy than her 14-year-old son who has had headaches off and on since he fell off his bicycle at age 8.

Although there are a few homeopathic remedies available over the counter that can be used to treat the occasional headache, people who suffer with frequent headaches, especially migraine, need professional help. I don't recommend trying to treat chronic headaches yourself; the choice of remedies available in the health food store is limited and choosing the wrong remedy will not bring the relief you seek.

That being said, many of the over-the-counter remedies have a particular pattern of headache pain and understanding a little about each remedy's headache symptom picture increases your ability to choose the remedy that fits.

ACONITUM NAPELLUS (ACONITE), BELLADONNA, and **GLONOINUM** are three remedies that have a very similar symptom presentation. The **headache** pattern for each of these remedies is **throbbing, bursting pain.** The head feels **hot and congested** as if the brain is too big for the skull. **Sudden onset** is a hallmark of each of these remedies as well. However, there are some unique, distinguishing characteristics that can help you choose which of these **throbbing** remedies to take or to offer to someone else.

Someone needing **ACONITE** will be much more **anxious** than someone who needs either **BELLADONNA** or **GLONOINUM**. **ACONITE** patients are so anxious they **fear** they are about to **have a stroke**

66

or might even **die**. The head feels **hot to the touch** and there is a marked feeling of **pressure in the forehead**.

The **BELLADONNA** patient typically has a **flushed, bright red face.** The headache is usually **worse on the right side** and **worse lying down.** The person needing **BELLADONNA** is extremely **sensitive to light, to noise, and to being jarred.** They prefer to **sit semi-erect** in a dark, quiet room and **prefer not to be touched.**

GLONIOINUM has one of the most rare and peculiar symptoms of all homeopathic remedies and I doubted such a thing existed until one of my patients presented with it. She described it this way, "I know you're going to think I'm crazy but every time I get a headache, I have this **feeling that my nose is disappearing**!" She would constantly ask her husband for reassurance that her nose was still its normal size and in its proper place on her face. Of course, not all people who need **GLONOINUM** will complain of this symptom but it is so classic for this remedy that its presence virtually guarantees that **GLONOINUM** is what is needed. **GLONOINUM** not only relieved her headaches but she no longer worries that she is losing her nose!

All three of these remedies can be used for **sunstroke** after prolonged sun exposure. The **ACONITE** patient will be extremely **anxious,** whereas the person needing **BELLADONNA** in this situation is more **delirious**. When the **veins of the temples** are **throbbing** and **distended**, **GLONOINUM** is the right remedy.

Give the appropriate remedy every 15 to 20 minutes on the way to the hospital. If you have only one of these remedies, in the event of **sunstroke,** give it. In an emergency situation, the remedies are close enough that giving whichever one you have is better than giving nothing while you wait for the paramedics. The risk of giving the wrong remedy is slight; the Vital Force is depleted and giving any of these three remedies will support it.

There is one other over-the-counter remedy that can be used for a headache with **throbbing, bursting pain. CHINA** has the peculiar symptom of a **headache that is relieved by nosebleeds.** Conversely it is also the remedy to consider when a **pulsating headache** comes on **after excessive menstrual bleeding.** In a **CHINA** headache, the pain usually affects the **temples** and the patient feels mentally **dull** and a bit **confused** as opposed to feeling **anxious** or **delirious.**

ALLERGY HEADACHES

As covered in the section on allergies, **ALLIUM CEPA,** made from red onion, is the first remedy to consider when there is a **burning sensation** in the eyes with lots of **tearing** as if you were chopping onions. A **dull headache over the forehead** that feels **worse in a warm, stuffy room** is another indication for **ALLIUM CEPA.** This remedy also has a very peculiar feature in that the **headache will stop with the onset of menstrual bleeding** and then **returns once the period is over.**

The headache associated with a cold or allergies where **EUPRHASIA** is the indicated remedy also tends to involve the **forehead.** However, rather than a dull ache, the **EUPHRASIA** headache has a feeling of **pressure** and **pulsation in the head.** There is also lots of **itching in the eyes**, with **tearing** and a large amount of **discharge from the nose. Sneezing** is also a hallmark symptom indicating the need for **EUPHRASIA** when headache is part of the allergy symptom picture.

HEADACHES IN CHILDREN

CALCAREA PHOSPHORICA is the classic remedy for **headaches in school-aged children**, especially around the time of **puberty**. You will recall this is the remedy to consider for **children with growing pains**. The headache pain tends to be **worse in the back of the skull** and also over the **bony sutures** at the top of the head. Often the child will complain that they can't hold their head up and you may notice their **head wobbles** a bit. **Throbbing pain in the forehead during menses,** especially in young women with chronic headaches, indicates the need for **CALC PHOS.**

This is not the only remedy useful for children with headaches. Any remedy that fits the entire symptom picture can be used for a child. With small children, I usually recommend starting with the 6c potency; if the relief is short-lived, you can always go up to the 30c potency.

EMOTIONAL HEADACHES

Headache is not uncommon during times of emotional stress. **ARGENTUM NITRICUM** and **IGNATIA AMARA** are two remedies available over the counter that often bring relief from **emotional turmoil. Anxiety** is one of the keynote symptoms of **ARGENTUM NITRICUM**. The 19th century language of the *Materia Medica* recommends this remedy for "headaches in hysterical young women and delicate literary persons" (Vermeulen's Concordant II). This is one of the first remedies to consider when a **migraine** develops **after an emotional shock or upset**, especially with a **feeling of panic.** The head can feel as if it is **in a vise** but oddly enough, **binding the head up with a tight cloth** actually makes the headache better.

Headache from acute grief is a common indication for **IGNATIA AMARA,** especially in women, although men benefit from this remedy as well. There is a *periodicity* to the **IGNATIA** headache, meaning the headaches can appear on a *regular basis* every week or at the same time of the month. The pain can feel *as if a nail were being driven* through the head, especially in the *forehead* and *above the eyes.*

One of the distinguishing features of the **IGNATIA** patient is that they are *very sensitive to tobacco smoke*, which makes all their complaints worse.

EYE STRAIN HEADACHES

RUTA GRAVEOLENS is very helpful for *eye strain*, especially from working at a computer or reading in dim light. The typical **RUTA** headache has *stitching or piercing pain* above the eyebrows and over the forehead.

The other over-the-counter remedy helpful for eye strain that causes headache is **PHOSPHORIC ACID**. The pain often involves the *top of the head* with a feeling of pressure. **PHOSPHORIC ACID** is also a common remedy for *overwhelming fatigue*; and is distinguished from **RUTA**, which has a tendency to *restlessness* rather than lassitude.

FLU HEADACHE

One of the first remedies to consider when you get a *headache at the onset of the flu* is **GELSEMIUM SEMPERVIRENS**. It's typically a dull headache that comes on **suddenly** with **body aches**. The pain can involve any part of the head but the key feature is its manifestation with **influenza**. **ACONITE** can also be used for a **sudden headache** that comes on at the beginning of an illness. But unlike **GELSEMIUM**, the **ACONITE** headache is usually associated with a cold or upper respiratory infection rather than the "ache-all-over" sensation that comes with the flu.

HEADACHES WITH GI SYMPTOMS

Four over-the-counter remedies have headaches that accompany symptoms in the gastrointestinal (GI) tract. Each remedy has a unique type of headache but they share one or all of the cardinal three symptoms that signal GI distress: **nausea, vomiting,** and **diarrhea.**

ARSENICUM ALBUM, as in the previous discussion of **food poisoning**, often has GI symptoms as one of its main signaling devices. Other hallmarks of **ARSENICUM** are **burning pain** and **restlessness.** The other peculiar symptom of an **ARSENICUM** *headache* is that **applying cold compresses to the head** brings relief even though the rest of the body may feel cold. **ARSENICUM** is another *periodic* remedy, meaning that the **symptoms tend to recur in a regular pattern**. So, someone who gets a **burning headache with GI symptoms** on a regular, recurrent basis that makes them toss and turn in bed and crave a cool washcloth on their forehead, most likely needs **ARSENICUM ALBUM.** Usually the 30c potency repeated every few hours brings relief after three or four doses if the remedy is correctly chosen.

71

CHELIDONIUM MAJUS is another remedy indicated when the Vital Force asks for help by producing **nausea, vomiting of bile,** and a **headache.** The headache of **CHELIDONIUM** often affects the **right side of the head** above the eye. The **pain can radiate** down the cheek and into the back of the head. The **back of the head** can feel **cold and heavy**. The other unusual feature indicating **CHELIDONIUM** is the **headache is better after eating**, even in the presence of nausea.

As a side note, **CHELIDONIUM** is often used to relieve pain from **gallstones** or **inflammation of the gallbladder**. A consultation with a homeopath can help determine if **CHELIDONIUM** is the right remedy for your gallbladder trouble. But for a simple **right-sided headache** with **nausea** and **vomiting bile,** it's worth trying **CHELIDONIUM** instead of acetaminophen or ibuprofen that tend to be hard on the GI tract.

Have you ever had a headache so bad that your hair hurt? **COLOCYNTHIS** has this symptom. Unlike **ARSENICUM** that **likes a cold cloth** on the head, the **COLOCYNTHIS headache is better from applying heat** to the head. The pain usually is located in **both temples**. **Lying on the back** makes the headache **worse**. The **face is often hot,** there may be a **glistening** quality to the **eyes** and the headache is often **better after drinking coffee**.

The last over-the-counter remedy for headaches with GI symptoms is **PODOPHYLLUM**, the remedy we learned about for **traveler's diarrhea**. **PODOPHYLLUM** has an unusual symptom in that the **headache alternates with diarrhea**. In other words, the headache temporarily disappears while the bowels are "letting loose" and then returns once the gut settles down. Remember, the **diarrhea** of **PODOPHYLLUM** is usually **yellow or green** and tends to come out in a **gush.** Taking this remedy not only relieves the headache, but it soothes the gut as well. The other prominent feature indicating that **PODOPHYLLUM** is the needed remedy is a **bitter taste in the mouth.**

HORMONAL HEADACHES

There are almost 400 remedies for headaches that occur due to **hormonal changes** or appear at various times **during the menstrual cycle.** Fortunately, the only one available over the counter is **SEPIA SUCCUS,** which is the quintessential hormonal remedy, especially well-suited for women.

SEPIA is made from the ink of the cuttlefish, the source of the brown pigment artists have used for centuries. It's a common remedy for women who get a **headache every time they have a menstrual period. SEPIA** is the first remedy to consider for women who develop **headaches during or after pregnancy.** During a **SEPIA** headache, the smell or taste of **food is repulsive.** The pain can be on only **one side of the head** and there can be **nausea and vomiting** as well. It's not so much the type of pain that distinguishes **SEPIA** from other headache remedies, as it is its **hormonal nature.**

HEADACHES FROM MENTAL EXERTION

There are three remedies available over the counter that can be very helpful when your **head hurts from thinking or studying too much**, especially if you are a student cramming for final exams. These are **CALCAREA CARBONICA, COFFEA CRUDA**, and **KALI PHOSPHORICUM. CALCAREA CARBONICA** has the unique feature of **headache with cold hands and feet**. The **head can feel cold** as well, especially on the right side, after too many hours of study or intense concentration.

The other keynote symptom of **CALCAREA** is **sweating of the head**, especially at the time of **menopause**.

COFFEA CRUDA can relieve **migraine**-type headache that comes on after drinking **too much coffee** and **hours of study**. Hours of thinking or talking over too many cups of coffee can bring on a headache that is **aggravated by light, noise, music, or smells.** The pain is usually a **throbbing pain about the temples** and **moving around makes it worse.** Lying in a dark, quiet room and taking **COFFEA CRUDA** every few hours can bring relief.

KALI PHOSPHORICUM, like its cousin **CALCAREA PHOSPHORICA**, is a remedy well suited to students. Whereas **CALC PHOS** has chronic **headaches and growing pains in children**, the headaches of **KALI PHOSPHORICUM** tend to occur after a session of **intense study and concentration**. People needing **KALI PHOS** tend to have **pain at the back of the head** and they are especially **sensitive to noise**. The other defining feature of a **KALI PHOS** headache is an **empty, hungry sensation** in the stomach. Gentle movement often makes the person needing **KALI PHOS** feel better.

MIGRAINE HEADACHES

There are about 60 remedies for migraine headaches cataloged in the *Materia Medica*; choosing the correct remedy usually requires professional homeopathic consultation. However, six of our over-the-counter remedies have **migraine** as part of their symptom picture.

Getting to know these remedies in advance may help you to figure out which one to try the next time migraine attacks.

NATRUM MURIATICUM is the sine qua non headache remedy. It is a classic remedy for headaches of all kinds, but especially *migraine headaches*. The feeling of a **NAT MUR** headache is "as if a thousand tiny hammers" were pounding on the head. Headaches that occur *after grief* or are worse from spending *time in the sun* often call for **NATRUM MURIATICUM**. The pain is usually *above the eyes* and there is often intense **photophobia** or *sensitivity to light*. People who need this remedy on a chronic basis often **crave salt** and will report that they have *never felt well since the loss of a loved one.*

Left-sided headaches with *bursting, throbbing pain*—especially if they start with the onset of *menopause*—call for **LACHESIS MUTA**. Made from the venom of the bushmaster snake, this remedy has an intensity to it that reflects its source. I personally took this remedy for several years when I developed high blood pressure. Taking this remedy under the supervision of my own homeopath spared me a lifetime of pharmaceutical drugs and my blood pressure is now completely normal. **LACHESIS** is a left-sided remedy; the headache usually starts on the left side and can radiate down into the jaw and the neck. During the time I had hypertension, I had a chronic ringing in the ears that went away after the course of **LACHESIS.** I have used this remedy successfully with many of my patients who developed *headaches* and *hot flashes* at the time of *menopause.* It's a powerful, deeply healing remedy and has many uses besides effectively treating *headache*.

A *word of caution:* do not try to treat yourself if you have *high blood pressure*. Although **LACHESIS** was the right remedy for me, there are about 170 remedies that can be used to treat hypertension. Consult a homeopath who is experienced in treating chronic conditions and knows how to help you make the transition from pharmaceutical drugs to homeopathic treatment without aggravating your condition.

As we touched on briefly when we mentioned *hangover*, **NUX VOMICA** is the first remedy to think of for *toxic headaches*. Like **BELLADONNA** and **GLONOINUM**, **NUX VOMICA** has *pounding, throbbing pain* in the head brought on by *drugs* of any kind, and especially after *excessive alcohol intake*. I routinely use it for almost all my clients *after general anesthesia*, which is a necessary, controlled kind of toxin. I usually recommend my postoperative patients take **NUX VOMICA** two to three times a day for a few days until all the effects of the anesthesia are gone.

Excessive irritability is one of the hallmarks of **NUX**. The other peculiar feature of someone presenting with a **NUX VOMICA** headache is the *desire to press his or her forehead against a hard surface.*

For migraine headaches that present with *overwhelming nausea* and *constant vomiting*, reach for **IPECACUANHA**. As we discussed in the section on *food poisoning*, **IPECACUANAHA**, made from ipecac, has a distinct feature: **intense vomiting** that brings no relief from the *nausea*. When intense vomiting that won't stop, even when there is nothing left in the stomach, comes on with onset of a migraine headache, **IPECACUANHA** can bring almost instant relief after just a few doses.

The next over-the-counter remedy that can be used for migraine headaches when the symptom picture fits is **BRYONIA**. This is one of my favorite remedies as I have used it many times to treat *migraine* *headaches* but also ***fungal pneumonia, bone fractures, and acute appendicitis WITHOUT SURGERY***. (You can read about that amazing case study in my first book.)

The hallmark symptom that calls for **BRYONIA** is *worse with motion.* In any complaint where the *slightest motion makes the patient feel horrible*, **BRYONIA** must be seriously considered. When **BRYONIA** is the remedy, the slightest movement of the eyeballs or any part of the head makes the migraine much worse. There can also be *nausea or other GI complaints* and the pain is often described as *splitting*, affecting any part of the head. Tying a bandanna or other cloth around the head may bring temporary relief but giving **BRYONIA** is the ultimate answer for *migraine headache worse with the slightest motion.*

The last of our over-the-counter migraine remedies is **SILICEA**, also called **SILICA**. The headache is usually located *over one eye* and has a *tendency to recur periodically*, especially after someone has recovered from a severe illness. Headaches that come on *after fasting* or from *skipping meals* often call for **SILICA**. Like most migraine sufferers, people needing **SILICA** prefer a dark quiet room. But the *cold air* especially *aggravates* **SILICA** patients and they like the room to be warm. Wrapping the head in a warm compress makes them feel better.

Interestingly, in the early days of homeopathy when traditional physicians were still trying to "balance the humors" by bloodletting and purging, they noticed that diuresis, or *profuse urination*, could relieve a **SILICA** headache. These days we just give **SILICA**, especially if the *fingernails are brittle* and *have white spots*, two of this remedy's distinguishing features.

SINUS HEADACHES

Although there are approximately 500 remedies that can be used in cases of **SINUS HEADACHE**, some of the more common ones indicated are available over the counter.

The remedy I find that works most often for **intense face pain** when the **sinuses are congested** is **KALI BICHROMICUM**. One of my patients calls this "the faucet remedy" because whenever she takes this for her sinus headache, her sinuses immediately start to drain. There is another closely related remedy in the same family called **KALI CARBONICUM** that is also very helpful in cases of **headache from sinus infection** or **allergies**. There are a few ways to tell these remedies apart.

KALI BICHROMICUM has **thick, tenacious, sticky**, **stringy, yellow mucus** that is hard to bring up. The discharge of **KALI CARBONICUM** is not as thick and it's not as difficult to expel. When a person needs **KALI CARB**, they tend to **sweat** more and they often complain of **backache** at the same time they have a **sinus headache**. Like **ACONITE, KALI CARB** can bring relief for people who get a **headache after being out in a cold wind** or riding in a convertible with the top down. **KALI CARB** patients also tend to **feel weak** when they get sick.

The **KALI BICH** headache tends to be more **intense, almost violent,** and there is a feeling as if the entire forehead is **one solid block**. The **nose is often stopped up** but will start to drain once the remedy is taken. The other distinguishing feature of **KALI BICH** is the **headache** is often **better after eating warm soup.**

There are two other over-the-counter remedies, also in the **KALI** family, that have unique features in addition to *sinus headache pain. Intense sinus pain over the eyes and root of the nose* with *severe tearing of the eyes* indicates the need for **KALI IODATUM**. There is often a sharp *pain in the forehead that is worse bending over. Hot, profuse, watery nasal discharge* with *intense tearing* and severe *sinus pressure in the forehead* is the classic presentation of **KALI IODATUM**.

Whereas thick, yellow mucus is a hallmark of sinusitis needing **KALI BICHROMICUM**, when the *mucus is thick but white* and the *tongue is coated white*, **KALI MURIATICUM** is the remedy to choose. *Vomiting thick, white phlegm* with lots of *sneezing* and *nasal discharge* also indicates this remedy.

Chronic recurring sinusitis, either from allergies or from chronic bacterial infection can be debilitating. Conventional medical treatment often requires multiple rounds of antibiotics year after year and expensive and painful surgery to "clean out" the sinuses. Over the years, I have seen countless patients get relief from homeopathic treatment, even after conventional drugs and surgery have failed to work.

Treating chronic sinus headaches homeopathically is fairly straightforward for a well-trained professional but can be daunting to try to treat on your own. But if you are serious about stopping the cycle of pain, antibiotics, and recurrent sinus surgeries, I highly recommend consulting an experienced, well-trained homeopathic professional. The treatment is less expensive than, and has none of the side effects of, conventional pharmaceutical drugs or surgery. Restoring the Vital Force to a state of health and balance, using well-chosen homeopathic remedies, makes it possible to never have another sinus headache again.

WEATHER HEADACHES

Headaches that occur with a change of weather or get worse during particular kinds of weather patterns are quite common. There are about 150 remedies where weather plays a role. The main over-the-counter remedy that has a distinct weather pattern is **PHOSPHORUS**. The peculiar feature of this remedy is the predisposition to develop a *headache before a thunderstorm*. There is also a marked *sensitivity to odors* and there can often be a feeling of profound *weakness. Dizziness* is often a common complaint with a headache needing **PHOSPHORUS.**

PHOSPHORUS is one of homeopathy's great remedies for *fatigue*. Taking **PHOSPHORUS** regularly, as with all "constitutional" remedies enhances the Vital Force's ability to achieve and maintain a state of health and well-being. Once the Vital Force is strengthened, long-standing or recurring symptoms like weather-related headaches disappear.

When I came to see Dr. Fry for a routine visit in December 2010, my body was covered with an extremely angry rash on my limbs and torso. I was beyond despair, having seen five dermatologists, an allergist, and an internist, none of whom had answers—only more tests and follow-up visits and numerous prescriptions which relieved the intense itching but didn't resolve the underlying cause. My issues were multifaceted: I was so fatigued during a normal workday that I would slip out to my car during the lunch hour to nap and I consumed energy drinks and caffeine to stay alert during the workday. Despite sleeping with a CPAP machine for sleep apnea, I would still feel exhausted throughout the day. I was so aggravated by allergies that I had resigned myself to staying indoors to avoid contact with trees and flowers.

After hearing my story in detail, Dr. Fry recommended a homeopathic remedy made from phosphorous. Interestingly, when I was young, our family moved to Florida when my father was hired to work on a long-term phosphorous extraction project and we lived in an area rich in natural phosphorous.

After taking the primary remedy, phosphorous, and another remedy, euphrasia, for my horrible allergies for several weeks, the angry red rash began to disappear. After about 6 months into homeopathic treatment, I felt very well. I was no longer exhausted and I could be outdoors without constantly sneezing and my eyes and ears no longer itched all the time.

Dr. Fry recommended another remedy, hypericum, for pain in my wrists and hands that had been diagnosed as carpal tunnel syndrome. My body had responded positively to each of the remedies and I finally had enough energy to get through the days and evenings without caffeine and energy drinks. It's great to have my life back, to have energy, and be in synch with life—a feeling I hadn't experienced for a long time. These are issues that had developed over a long time and weren't resolved overnight, but I'm thankful that I stuck with the program and I have now reaped the rewards. The rash went away completely and has never returned. I rarely suffer with allergies and when I do, I know which remedy to take. I am pain free and I have plenty of energy to do all the things I love to do. And I no longer have to take pharmaceutical drugs.

HEAD INJURY

Any head injury serious enough to need homeopathic treatment requires professional attention. The two main remedies available over the counter to give immediately on the way to seeking professional help are **ARNICA MONTANA** and **NATRUM SULPHURICUM.**

ARNICA is the number one remedy in nearly all cases of *trauma*, not just in *head injury*. In cases of *concussion, whiplash,* or *falls involving the head and neck*, giving **ARNICA** immediately can help prevent complications at a later date. In minor falls, the 30c potency repeated every few hours until all the symptoms have subsided is usually sufficient. However, in severe cases such as *concussions* or *injuries sustained in motor vehicle accidents*, the 200c potency is often needed. The rule of thumb is the more intense the experience, the higher the potency that is needed and the more often it should be repeated.

ARNICA MONTANA also has a very distinct symptom in that invariably the patient *insists there is nothing wrong with them,* even in cases where it is obvious to any observer that they are seriously injured. I distinctly remember a patient I was assigned to follow when I was a medical student on my first cardiology rotation. He had been admitted the night before from the Emergency Department after his wife brought him in because he had been complaining of chest pain and sweating profusely. His EKG showed that there was substantial damage to his heart muscle, that is, that he had suffered a heart attack.

But he insisted to anyone and everyone that there was nothing wrong with him and that he needed to get back to work!

Many years later when I first started my homeopathic studies, I remembered him when reading about this classic symptom of **ARNICA MONTANA:** "Sends the doctor away, insists that he is well." Although we think of **ARNICA** primarily as a remedy for trauma to the external body, clearly it can and should be used in cases of trauma to the internal organs such as the heart or lungs, especially if the patient insists there is nothing wrong despite clear evidence to the contrary.

NATRUM SULPHURICUM is the classic remedy to consider after *falls or blows to the head resulting in injury. Chronic headaches* that started after a head injury often indicate the need for **NAT SULPH.** *Mental symptoms* such as *depression, anxiety,* or *irritability* can also appear after head injury when this remedy is needed. Intense *sensitivity to sunlight* or *photophobia* is another symptom pointing to **NATRUM SULPHURICUM.**

Both of these remedies are commonly used by homeopaths to treat chronic conditions of various kinds where the common denominator is that their onset occurred after a serious head injury or trauma.

HEARTBURN AND INDIGESTION

Heartburn is a generic term that can mean different things to different people. The common medical term is gastroesophageal reflux disorder, or GERD. This simply describes the backing up of acidic fluid from the stomach into the esophagus. Conventional medical therapy usually involves prescribing medications to either neutralize the stomach acid or to stop its production with a class of drugs known as proton pump inhibitors, such as "the purple pill."

In homeopathic medicine, we take a different approach in that we are more concerned with uncovering the reason that the Vital Force is deranged and producing symptoms specific to the gut. Although there are more than 400 remedies for heartburn and indigestion listed in the *Materia Medica*, this section focuses on the more commonly used remedies available to most people over the counter.

The section on **COLDS** covered a remedy called **ANTIMONIUM TARTARICUM** that primarily affects the respiratory tract. **ANTIMONIUM CRUDUM** is a related remedy but its symptoms are centered mostly in the GI tract. People needing **ANTIMONIUM CRUDUM, or ANT-C,** will describe having a sensitive stomach. Their *digestion is easily disturbed* and they often reach for antacids after they eat. They frequently complain that their *stomach always feels full* and their food won't digest properly. The *tongue* usually has a *thick white coating.*

Bread and pastry are particularly *aggravating* and this remedy can be helpful for those who may be gluten intolerant. One of the unusual symptoms of this remedy is a *sweetish taste to the "waterbrash,"* the 19th century term for reflux.

The other prominent symptom indicating **ANTIMONIUM CRUDUM** is *constant belching.* This remedy is also helpful for babies who constantly spit up or *vomit after nursing*. Dissolve the 6c pellet in water and give the baby a teaspoonful of the remedy at feeding time to help settle the stomach and improve digestion.

CHELIDONIUM MAJUS is one of those remedies that is often overlooked but has the power to help the Vital Force when the liver and gallbladder are the areas crying out for help. The classic symptom that always makes me consider this remedy is ***pain in the stomach or abdomen that radiates through to the right shoulder blade***. This is the classic presentation of gallbladder colic caused by inflammation of the gallbladder with or without gallstones.

I have seen this remedy successfully help patients to pass gallstones and to spare them from gallbladder surgery. **CHELIDONIUM** patients are often ***incredibly irritable***; the slightest thing sets them off. They also have a lot of ***burping*** and ***belching. Nausea and vomiting of bile***, the bitter tasting fluid made in the gallbladder, is common and **CHELIDONIUM** can ease this as well.

It's important to make a distinction between the homeopathic and herbal preparation of **CHELIDONIUM**, also known as Greater Celandine. Remember that the homeopathic remedy is made by serially diluting a mother tincture of the concentrated herb. In this way, the *healing energy* of the plant is captured and held in sugar pellets.

In herbal medicine, the plant itself is taken directly in either tincture or pill form or brewed as a tea. There have been cases of *liver toxicity* reported in the medical literature from people taking Greater Celandine in herbal form for various skin conditions or to detoxify the liver.

However, taking the homeopathic preparation has none of the toxicity associated with the raw plant because once the mother tincture has been diluted and succussed to the 12c potency, virtually no molecules of the original plant remain.

It is initially hard for us to get our heads around the concept that something so dilute can be so powerful. However, the proof is in the pudding, so to speak, and those of us who have benefitted from homeopathic remedies become loyal advocates for their use.

Treating gallstones and gallbladder colic requires professional help but this is one of the remedies most commonly used by homeopaths and it's very helpful to have on hand for nausea and pain when the gallbladder or liver is irritated and inflamed.

As discussed earlier in the section on hangover, **NUX VOMICA** is the quintessential remedy for ailments from "high living." It's usually the first remedy to take for garden variety heartburn or indigestion brought on by drinking too much *coffee* or *alcohol* and/or eating too much *spicy food*.

One of my patients absolutely loves very spicy Mexican food served with a cold margarita. Before he started homeopathic treatment, he would have to take over-the-counter antacids and reflux drugs before and after his favorite meal. Once he started regular, constitutional treatment with **NUX VOMICA**, he could eat his favorite foods without having to take antacids. Interestingly, the intense craving for spicy foods and tequila lessened and his irritability improved as well.

NUX VOMICA patients also tend to be very irritable, usually because they have been *working too hard* and not getting enough rest and exercise. Almost every successful business person I have treated in my practice has needed this remedy at some time during their course of treatment. *Indigestion after business anxiety* should always bring **NUX VOMICA** to mind.

Pl. XLIV.

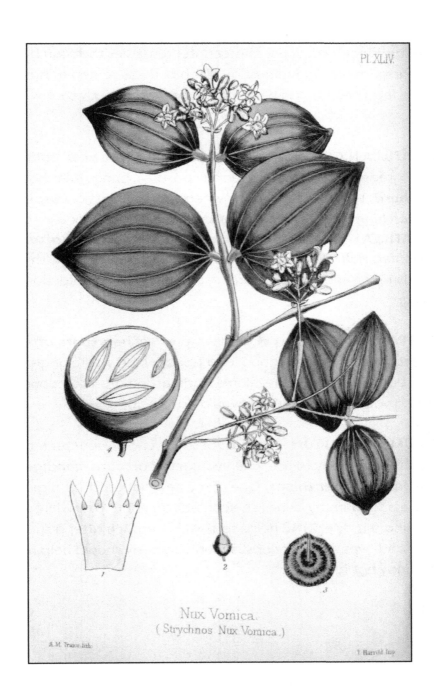

Nux Vomica.
(Strychnos Nux Vomica.)

A.M. Trazor. lith.

T. Harrold Imp

87

There are three other over-the-counter remedies that can be used for heartburn and/or indigestion. Each of these remedies has a unique feature that can help you choose the remedy that will work best for your particular type of heartburn.

PULSATILLA NIGRICANS is the remedy to think of when eating very rich or greasy, fatty foods, especially pastries, brings on a bout of *heartburn*. Think of this remedy when you have lots of *burping* and *belching* where *the taste of the food persists* for a long time. **PULSATILLA** is helpful when your *clothes feel too tight after eating something rich* (like cheesecake). You'll learn more about this remedy in the sections on morning sickness and ear infections in children.

STAPHYSAGRIA has the peculiar symptom of *heartburn after indignation.* It's never a good idea to eat when you're angry or upset but if you've ever developed indigestion after someone insulted you, **STAPHYSAGRIA** would have helped.

ZINCUM METALLICUM is the last of the over-the-counter remedies and it's the remedy to use when you get *heartburn or indigestion from eating sweet things.* One of my new patients has a great fondness for gummy bears; she can eat an entire bag while watching a movie. **ZINC** helps settle her stomach after a sugar binge and over time her constitutional remedy should help her break the candy habit.

HEMORRHOIDS

If you're someone who suffers from painful swelling of hemorrhoidal tissue, there are two over-the-counter homeopathic alternatives to conventional creams and suppositories. Bear with me as we discuss a particularly sensitive subject. Hemorrhoids, or piles as our grandparents called them, are actually swollen blood vessels located in the lower rectum and anus. Hemorrhoids are caused by an increase in pressure in the veins usually as a result of pregnancy or from straining to pass stool due to constipation.

There are two kinds of hemorrhoids: internal or external. Internal hemorrhoids are located inside the anus or rectum and rarely cause pain. Most people don't know they have them until they notice blood on the outside of the stool or blood dripping into the toilet after a bowel movement.

External hemorrhoids are located on the outside of the anus and can usually be seen and felt. They tend to be more painful but can also bleed especially from bearing down during a bowel movement. This type of hemorrhoid is also more likely to develop a thrombosis where a blood clot forms inside the vessel. This can be especially painful and may require surgery.

There can be other more serious causes of rectal bleeding, including colorectal cancer. A change in the size or color of stool can also be warning signs of cancer. Melena, or black stools, is a sign of bleeding higher up in the rectum or colon. If you have *any* of these symptoms, you should see your doctor or health care professional immediately.

Once you know that it is just hemorrhoids, there are a few remedies available over the counter that can bring relief.

AESCULUS HIPPOCASTUNUM is the remedy to take for *external hemorrhoids that are swollen and usually purple.* **HAMAMELIS VIRGINIANA** is especially helpful for *bleeding hemorrhoids*. **HAMAMELIS** can be used for all kinds of *bleeding* with sometimes dramatic results. Years ago, I had two surgical patients who developed bleeding in their incision about 1 week postoperatively. I happened to be out of town at a homeopathic conference and my nurse practitioner, Mary, called me very concerned. Both patients presented within a few hours of each other bleeding from their incision sites and none of the usual techniques, like pressure and cautery with silver nitrate, were working.

Coincidentally, we had just been studying the remedy **HAMAMELIS** and I knew right away the remedy that my patients needed. Fortunately, we had some in the office and Mary gave both of the patients a dose of the 30c potency. She repeated the remedy every 15 minutes and after three doses the bleeding stopped completely. As it turns out, there had been a bad batch of suture at the hospital. Surgical sutures are treated in a special way so they will begin to dissolve or be absorbed by the body after about 6 weeks. In these cases, the suture began to melt after only 1 week. Fortunately, **HAMAMELIS** stopped the bleeding and Steri-Strips® with pressure bandages saved these patients from a trip back to the OR.

Incidentally, the other remedy I had them take was **STAPHYSAGRIA** because it *promotes wound healing*. I often recommend **STAPHYSAGRIA** for my surgical patients for several reasons. Not only does it speed wound healing, it can be used in place of prophylactic antibiotics to *prevent wound infections*. It is the classic remedy to take for *pain or infection in the bladder* from a urinary catheter used during surgery.

Both **AESCULUS** and **HAMAMELIS** can be very helpful in relieving pain and bleeding when hemorrhoids flare up. Increasing fiber in the diet, especially from flaxseed, and drinking more water can prevent constipation that aggravates hemorrhoids. However, thrombosed or persistent, bleeding hemorrhoids require professional help.

PODOPHYLLUM is one of the remedies available over the counter to help pregnant women who suffer with hemorrhoids. This is a common complaint in pregnancy as the weight of the baby creates back pressure in the veins of the rectum and anus. **PODOPHYLLUM** can help bleeding and painful swelling from *hemorrhoids that have prolapsed,* or protruded, from the anal canal.

HOARSENESS (see COLDS)

INSECT BITES

The first remedy to take for any kind of insect bite, even bee stings, is **LEDUM PALUSTRE.** Homeopathically prepared from wild rosemary, **LEDUM** is the must-have remedy for *any kind of puncture.* It is commonly used *to prevent tetanus* after stepping on a nail, for example. It can also be used for pain at the site of any injection or vaccination. Pain that persists after dental work with multiple injections of Novocain® is a perfect setting for **LEDUM.**

A wasp stung me while I was watering my tomatoes and the pain was instant and intense. I immediately took **LEDUM** and within seconds the pain was gone. The pain came back after about 20 minutes and went away again when I took another dose. I took a total of four doses of LEDUM over the course of a few hours, completely stopping the pain and preventing any swelling.

I recommend this remedy for all my clients when they travel. Many years ago, I was traveling with a friend in Mexico who stepped on a stingray. The stinger got stuck in his foot and required a visit to a rather sketchy clinic on the beach, as I didn't have any medical instruments with me. The sting was very painful and his foot swelled so badly that he could barely walk for the next few days. If only I had known about **LEDUM!**

The other remedy my friend needed that day for the swelling was **APIS MELLIFICA. APIS** is prepared homeopathically from a mother tincture prepared from a whole honeybee, including the stinger. Most people assume that you should give **APIS** immediately for a bee sting. However, the first remedy to give is **LEDUM** for the effects of the puncture. **APIS** is indicated primarily if there is *redness* and *swelling*. As in the discussion of allergies, **APIS** is the remedy to consider when there is swelling of any kind.

APIS is often used by professional homeopaths in the treatment of *blood clots* in the legs where there is substantial *redness* and *swelling*. This is not something you should try at home but it is good to know that by consulting a professional homeopathic practitioner

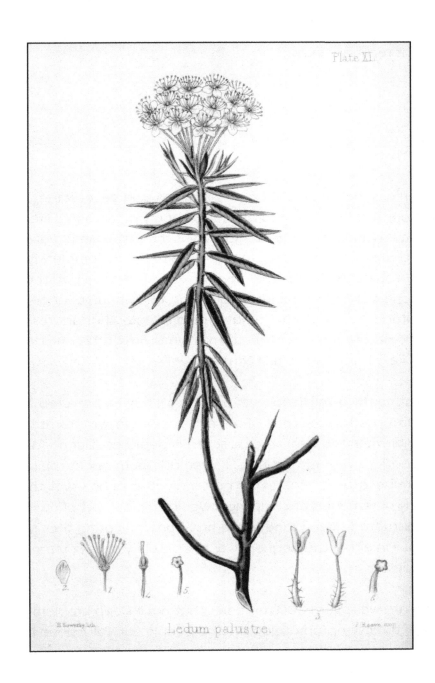

Plate XI.

H Sowerby lith.

Ledum palustre.

J Reeve imp.

93

you may be able to avoid taking blood-thinning medications and prevent recurrent clots.

INSOMNIA

Insomnia is the symptom that made me a true believer in homeopathy and changed the course of my professional life and practice. Twenty-nine years ago, I went through a period of stress and I couldn't sleep to save my life despite being completely exhausted at the end of the day. The fatigue was so bad that I postponed all my scheduled surgeries, took a short vacation, and consulted a homeopath. He gave me a remedy that addressed my specific situation and covered all my symptoms. After one dose, I slept like a baby for the first time in weeks.

In treating my own clients over the years, I have discovered that disrupted sleep is one of the most common symptoms that presents when the Vital Force is severely depleted. During follow-up consultations with my patients, I often ask them about their sleep pattern because it's one of the best indicators of how well their remedy or remedies are working. I would say for most of my clients, that disrupted sleep is one of the first clues indicating they need an increase in either the frequency or the potency of their remedy or remedies.

There are well over 1,000 remedies that have sleep problems as part of their symptomatology. Some people can fall asleep but have trouble staying asleep. In my experience, most people have a combination of both symptoms. Oftentimes, something will awaken them during the night and then they can't go back to sleep because their mind is overstimulated. Vivid dreams or nightmares can also disrupt sleep and make it difficult to fall back asleep.

Obviously, chronic or severe insomnia as in my case requires the skill of a professional homeopath. However, for occasional bouts of insomnia due to emotional shock, grief, overwork, or too much coffee, there are several over-the-counter remedies worth trying first.

RESTLESS SLEEP

Of the 20 or so over-the-counter remedies that have insomnia as part of their symptom picture, six of these have **restlessness during sleep. ACONITUM NAPELLUS** has **restless sleep during a febrile illness**. Taking **ACONITE** often relieves insomnia after any kind of **shock** or from **fear**. This remedy is very helpful for **insomnia in the elderly.** People needing **ACONITE** will often have **anxious dreams** that cause them to toss and turn in bed.

ARSENICUM ALBUM is another restless sleep remedy but people needing this remedy commonly **awaken between 1 and 3 am**. They often have trouble falling asleep because they are **anxious** or **in pain. Dreams about people who have died** are a common symptom indicating **ARSENICUM.** One distinguishing factor between **ACONITE** and **ARSENICUM** is body temperature; **ARSENICUM** is a "chilly" remedy, whereas people needing **ACONITE** when they can't sleep tend to be hot, especially when they are sick.

BELLADONNA is another hot, restless remedy but it is a **short-acting** remedy, meaning that it's not usually indicated for people with long-standing, chronic insomnia. **BELLADONNA** is helpful for *restless sleep in children with high fever* whose *skin is hot*. Remember this is the *red cheeks* remedy.

There is an intensity about **BELLADONNA** that can manifest with *crying out* or even *screaming during sleep*. *Frightful dreams* or *nightmares* causing frequent waking throughout the night call for **BELLADONNA**. This is another *must-have* remedy for parents of small children. It can rapidly reduce a fever that comes on suddenly during the night and help bring sleep to a restless, crying child in pain. During the swine flu epidemic several years back, this remedy was invaluable for helping my patients who had very high fevers that kept them from getting the sleep they sorely needed.

I once treated another patient with this remedy who had a symptom peculiar to **BELLADONNA:** every time she had a fever from a sinus infection she would have *dreams of fire.*

As expected from a remedy made from unroasted coffee beans, **COFFEA CRUDA** is another remedy very well suited to those who can't sleep, especially after a day of *excessive coffee drinking*. **COFFEA** not only helps people who can't fall asleep, it also helps people fall back to sleep after waking in the middle of the night. Unlike the other restless sleep remedies (**ACONITE, ARSENICUM, BELLADONNA), COFFEA** *dreams* are often *pleasant* and *happy*.

The section on anxiety discusses the remedy **GELSEMIUM SEMPERVIRENS** for its ability to calm nervous fliers. It is also helpful for not being able to sleep due to *exhaustion*. The restlessness associated with this remedy is often *worse toward the morning.* Sleep disturbance of any kind associated with **flu** is often helped by **GELSEMIUM.**

ZINCUM METALLICUM is the remedy to take for sleep that's disrupted from frequent *cramps in the legs* or from *restless leg syndrome.* This remedy is also helpful, especially in the elderly, when there's *a feeling of bugs crawling up the legs.* Obviously that sensation makes sleep almost impossible. Like the remedy **CHINA, ZINC** is helpful when *cold feet* wake you up in the middle of the night.

<u>**UNREFRESHING SLEEP**</u>

No one expects to feel great after a night spent tossing and turning in bed. However, there are many cases when people will sleep most of the night but don't feel refreshed when they awaken in the morning. There are remedies that can help the Vital Force recover from certain stressors that can lead to feeling "wiped out" rather than well rested in the morning.

COCCULUS INDICUS is the primary remedy for ailments from *night watching.* If you have ever sat up most of the night caring for an ill child (or delivering a baby, as I did for many years), you know that horrible feeling of being completely drained. When this happens night after night, the Vital Force really takes a hit. **COCCULUS** is the ideal remedy for *depleted caregivers* who are on their last nerve.

It's not just the sleeplessness that can put people into a **COCCULUS** state. The kind of worry and anxiety you see in parents keeping vigil over their premature baby in the NICU (neonatal intensive care unit) coupled with lack of sleep instigates the need for this remedy. **COCCULUS** patients wake up wishing they could just stay in bed for the entire day because they are *exhausted.* They are *very irritable* and the slightest thing sets them off, especially *noise.*

97

Many a medical student or resident putting in long hours caring for very sick patients have needed this remedy over the years. People who need **COCCULUS** will often complain they feel so depleted that everything slows down. Their thinking slows down and so does their reaction time. They are so exhausted, it takes them longer to do the simplest of tasks.

I recommend taking the 30c potency in the morning. You may need an extra dose at bedtime for a while until your vitality returns. For professional caregivers, this remedy may be needed long term in increasing potency over time, as the 30c potency may not be strong enough. A professional homeopath can give you guidance on how often and how long to take this remedy and where to get the higher potencies.

I'm not sure which of our homeopathic predecessors first coined the expression but **CHINA OFFICINALIS** is known for *building air castles*. This is a quaint 19th century expression describing folks who lie in bed at night and can't sleep because they are *making lots of plans* and spinning fantasies in their head all night. Of course, they will wake up feeling exhausted and sometimes have a headache.
This is a good remedy for *busy multitaskers* who can't seem to shut their minds off when it's time for bed. You will recall this is also the remedy for people who develop *fatigue from loss of vital fluids.* It's not uncommon for women with abnormally heavy menstrual flow to need **CHINA** to relieve the insomnia that often occurs during their periods. **CHINA** is also one of the remedies when *cold feet* awaken one from sleep.

LACHESIS has the peculiar symptom of *sleeping into an aggravation*, meaning that all their complaints are *worse after a night's sleep. Headaches, menstrual cramps, or high blood* *pressure* are some of the **LACHESIS** conditions that are *worse in the morning*. People needing **LACHESIS** often *awaken tired* as well. It's a remedy especially well-suited to *sleeplessness in alcoholics.* **NATRUM MURIATICUM** is another over-the-counter remedy that can help people who *awaken feeling tired.* Remember that **NAT MUR** is a common remedy for people suffering from *grief*, which can certainly disturb one's sleep. Persons needing this remedy often lie in bed at night ruminating about *things that have happened in the past*, which keeps them from falling asleep. *Frequent jerking of the limbs* during sleep is also a hallmark of this remedy. *Sleepwalking* is also a common symptom for people who need **NAT MUR**.

IGNATIA AMARA is the other over-the-counter remedy that is helpful for people who suffer with *insomnia after suffering grief.* In fact, **NATRUM MURIATICUM** is the chronic option. In cases of acute *grief where there is prolonged crying and inability to sleep,* **IGNATIA** is the remedy. In some cases, the grief is deep, buried, and prolonged; this often occurs when someone needed **IGNATIA** at the time of the death of a loved one but never got it. The symptom of grief then becomes chronic and **IGNATIA** is not as helpful. In these cases, **NATRUM MURIATICUM** is the remedy to give, especially when *headaches develop after untreated grief.*

IGNATIA in general is a very helpful remedy for people who often manifest *emotional symptoms* when under stress. As expected, sleep can be disrupted when someone is having relationship troubles that have him or her very upset. People needing **IGNATIA** to treat their insomnia tend to be *overwrought* and a bit *dramatic* about circumstances in their lives that often seem out of proportion to others around them.

SILICA, made from flint, can be very helpful for people who are **sleepy all day,** because they don't get a night of deep, refreshing sleep. **SILICA** is helpful for people who feel **sleepy after eating.** They also tend to awaken **frequently** and to **talk in their sleep.**

OTHER CAUSES OF INSOMNIA

In my experience, it's not uncommon for people who generally sleep well every night to develop insomnia under certain circumstances. Several of the over-the-counter remedies can help restore sleep disrupted by specific causes. For example, **CHAMOMILLA** is a godsend for parents when their baby cannot sleep due to **pain from teething or from ear infections.** Place one pellet of the remedy in water and give the baby a teaspoonful before bedtime. You may need to repeat it again through the night if baby awakens again in pain.

Children who suffer from **night terrors** benefit greatly from **CALCAREA CARBONICA.** Often children will complain of **dreaming about monsters** that waken them in a panic. This is also a good remedy for people who can't fall asleep at night because they are **worried** about something. I have found this remedy very helpful for people who are sick and constantly **worry they will never be well again.**

One of the symptoms that distinguishes **CALCAREA** from some of the other worrying remedies like **IGNATIA** or **NUX VOMICA** is **sweating.** People who need **CALCAREA** sweat very easily, especially about the head. This is a common symptom in menopausal women who awaken with hot flashes and night sweats, as shown a bit later in this book.

Insomnia due to coughing is a common symptom calling for the remedy **KALI CARBONICUM.** (See sinus headaches.)

DROSERA ROTUNDIFOLIA is another remedy for *coughing that is worse lying down at night* (see colds). Unlike **DROSERA,** people who need **KALI CARB** tend to *talk in their sleep.* Between the coughing and the talking, it's no wonder folks needing this remedy can't sleep!

As in the section on hangovers, **NUX VOMICA** is the quintessential remedy for people who eat or drink too much or abuse drugs. *Insomnia after a heavy night of partying* calls for **NUX VOMICA** and helps to avoid the pain from a hangover the next morning. Hard-driving, irritable businesspeople who self-medicate with drugs and alcohol benefit greatly from **NUX VOMICA.** One of my clients is a very successful chief executive of an international corporation and **NUX VOMICA** has been a lifesaver for him during periods of severe stress. He recently told me that he didn't think he would have been able to keep working, much less sleeping well, without the support of this remedy.

Dreams of various kinds can disrupt sleep and make it difficult to go back to sleep. One over-the-counter remedy in particular is very helpful for people who *weep in their sleep due to sad dreams.* That remedy is **PULSATILLA,** a common remedy for children. They tend to have a hard time getting up in the morning and prefer to sleep in late. *Whining* both in their sleep and while awake is one of the keynote symptoms of **PULSATILLA.**

The last over-the-counter remedy that has a peculiar feature of insomnia is **RHUS TOXICODENDRON.** As we shall see a little later in joint pain discussion, **RHUS TOX** is a common remedy for people who awaken in the morning with *stiff joints.* The peculiar thing about their sleep, however, is that they will have *dreams of great exertion* and awaken stiff and sore. One of my clients repeatedly dreamed she was running the Boston marathon every night and she would wake up so sore she couldn't get out of bed without taking ibuprofen first. And she wasn't even a runner!

LEG AND MUSCLE CRAMPS

There are two over-the-counter homeopathic remedies listed for use for muscle cramps: **CUPRUM METALLICUM** and **ZINCUM METALLICUM.** Although both remedies are made from minerals and have muscle cramps as part of their symptom picture, there are a few distinguishing features that can help you decide which remedy to take for muscle cramps.

The muscle cramps calling for **CUPRUM** usually involve the calves of the legs, the soles of the feet, and the palms of the hands. The muscles go into spasm and can be quite painful. The cramps in the palms can be so severe that the thumbs turn inward in a clench.

ZINC is a much more *restless* remedy and in the homeopathic provings, it affected the *feet* primarily. As discussed in the section on insomnia, this remedy can be helpful for *restless leg syndrome*, especially when the feet are the most involved.

MENOPAUSAL SYMPTOMS

After 30 years of caring for women in obstetrics and gynecology and as a homeopath, I would venture to say that I have heard probably every variation on the theme of hot flashes associated with menopause. When prescribing conventional hormone therapy, the timing, intensity, and location of the hot flashes doesn't matter—most every woman gets a variation of some kind of either bioidentical or synthetic estrogen with or without progesterone.

Choosing the correct homeopathic remedy to stop the flushing, sweating, and attendant sleep disruption and mood changes requires attention to the details of each woman's unique story. Each woman will need a different remedy depending on how her symptoms manifest.

The *Materia Medica* lists 80 remedies for "flushes of heat in the climacteric period"; although most women will find relief from one of these remedies, there are only six that are available over the counter. Even with this limited number of choices available to you, it's worth trying one of these remedies especially if you can't or don't want to take hormone therapy.

I would recommend choosing the remedy that most closely fits your symptoms and try the 30c potency once a day for a few weeks. If you don't notice any relief at all, try a different remedy. I'll do my best to give you a clear symptom picture of each of the over-the-counter remedies available for you to try. Avoiding coffee and strong mint will give the remedy the best chance of working. In most cases, you will need increasing potencies of the remedy over time and that usually requires a consultation with a homeopath on how and when to make an adjustment. But many women find taking the 30c potency daily is sufficient to bring relief and enables them to avoid conventional hormone therapy.

Women often ask me how long they will need to take the remedy. I tell them that there is no set formula and that every woman's needs are different. In general, if you have chosen the right remedy, your symptoms will abate and the relief will usually last 6 to 8 weeks. If and when the symptoms return, try taking the remedy twice a day—that may bring relief for another month or so. If it doesn't, you will need a higher potency. Each increase in potency will usually bring relief.

Higher potencies will usually bring relief that lasts for a longer period of time, sometimes even for several months. However, when you no longer need the remedy, your symptoms will return and going up to the next potency only makes them worse. This indicates that you are proving the remedy and it's time to stop. The symptoms will usually disappear in a day or two, indicating you are finished with this remedy. If the symptoms don't go away, you either need a different remedy or there is something interfering with the action of the remedy. At this point, I would recommend consulting a professional homeopath for further guidance.

BELLADONNA is the first remedy to consider for *hot flashes that come on suddenly* and turn your *face bright red. Sweating* is common, especially on the chest, but unlike **CALCAREA,** the head is dry. When women need **BELLADONNA** during menopause, they notice that they are very *irritable* and everything and everyone irritates them. Although **BELLADONNA** is typically a remedy for short-lived illnesses like **fever due to ear infections,** I have used it in increasing potencies over several years for menopausal women.

CALCAREA CARBONICA is the first remedy to think of when you've got your makeup perfectly done and the **sweat comes pouring down your head and face.** This is the remedy for sweating so severely that you have to change your pajamas and/or the sheets on the bed in the middle of the night. (Very disruptive for your sleeping partner, too!) Whereas women needing **BELLADONNA** feel irritable, women who benefit from **CALCAREA** often complain of **feeling exhausted from overwork** or **overwhelmed from too much responsibility. CALCAREA** women tend to be **worriers,** especially about their loved ones. They can also be more **anxious about their health** and worry about getting diseases like Alzheimer's or Parkinson's.

As discussed in the section on headaches, **GLONOINUM** is a **throbbing remedy** that has an intense energy about it, which makes sense considering that it's made from nitroglycerine. **Intense flushes of heat affecting the head,** especially with a headache, call for **GLONOINUM.** Like **BELLADONNA** the face can be bright red but when **GLONOINUM** is needed, the headache is much more intense and the veins of the temple are often distended and pulsating.

In my experience, these two remedies are so similar that it can be hard to know which one to choose. If you're not sure which of these two remedies is correct, start with **BELLADONNA 30c** once a day. If you don't notice any change after several days, switch to the **GLONOINUM.** If you're suffering with a pounding headache, you may need to repeat the remedy every few hours until it abates. As always, if you don't get relief from either of these remedies even though they match your symptoms closely, consult a professional (see headaches).

LACHESIS MUTA is one of the remedies I recommend most frequently in my practice for women during menopause. Most women complain of hot flashes that begin in the core of the body and radiate out to the arms and legs. Sweating is not as intense as it is with **CALCAREA** but **LACHESIS** has some distinct features that set it apart from other menopausal remedies. Women needing **LACHESIS** will often complain of *heart palpitations* where the pulse races and the *heart beat increases during a hot flash*. Unlike women needing **SEPIA** (see below), the *sex drive is increased* when the Vital Force is asking for **LACHESIS.** The question I often ask women when I'm trying to determine if **LACHESIS** is their remedy is, "How do you feel when you wear a turtleneck sweater?" **LACHESIS** people will emphatically tell you they hate them because they *can't stand wearing any type of tight clothing* around the neck or the waist. They may also have a *fear of snakes.*

Another interesting feature of **LACHESIS** is that it is *a left-sided remedy,* meaning that symptoms often primarily affect the left side of the body. One of my clients suffered for years with ringing in her left ear only. Once she started **LACHESIS** for her menopausal symptoms, the ear ringing stopped completely and never returned. I find this left sidedness especially interesting given the source of this remedy. **LACHESIS MUTA** is made from the venom of the bushmaster snake, one of the deadliest snakes in South America. And when it eats its prey, its jaw disarticulates (comes apart), starting on the left side.

The last two over-the-counter remedies that are helpful for menopausal women are **IGNATIA** and **SEPIA.**

As in the section on anxiety, **IGNATIA** is a remedy whose action is primarily in the emotional sphere. Women needing this remedy at the time of menopause don't suffer from hot flashes and night sweats so much. The most prominent symptoms are emotional, especially so if women experience grief around the time of menopause.

I once treated a patient who came into my office sobbing uncontrollably. She could hardly get out the words to tell me what was wrong. Finally, she was able to calm herself enough to tell me that her husband of 27 years had just left her for his secretary. She never saw it coming and the shock of it was so severe that in addition to nonstop crying, she hadn't been able to sleep for several days and she had very heavy menstrual bleeding for the first time in 9 months. A pelvic exam and pelvic ultrasound were normal. I recommended **IGNATIA AMARA** 30c daily and within a few days, the bleeding stopped and never returned.

It took another few weeks before she could sleep through the night. Although the crying subsided, she was still quite emotional. She sought counseling with the pastor of her church and that helped her as well. She took **IGNATIA** for the better part of 2 years while she went through the divorce and eventually she was able to stop it once she recovered her emotional equilibrium. In my experience, this remedy is a much healthier alternative for my patients than prescribing habit-forming tranquilizers like Valium® or Xanax® because it treats the cause of the symptoms, which is always an imbalance in the Vital Force, our innate inner healer.

Your situation is hopefully not quite as dramatic. But if you find that you are more emotional than usual as your menses begin to dwindle, **IGNATIA** may be the remedy you need, especially if you're grieving a loss.

SEPIA SUCCUS is the sine qua non remedy for hormonal complaints. It is traditionally thought of as a woman's remedy because it primarily affects the hormonal system. But the very first self-proving of a remedy occurred in a gentleman who was a patient of Dr. Samuel Hahnemann, the 18th century German physician who discovered, researched, and codified the principles that formed the foundation for homeopathic medicine.

The story goes that Dr. Hahnemann was caring for a gentleman with numerous complaints. Dr. Hahnemann tried a number of remedies but nothing seemed to work. So, he made a house call in order to observe the patient in his own environment and see if something there could give him a clue as to what the remedy might be.

As it happens, the patient was a painter and he was using cuttlefish ink as paint. Dr. Hahnemann watched him as he would lick the paintbrush, dip it into the ink, and lick the brush again. Hahnemann realized that the man was slowly being poisoned by repeatedly dosing himself with squid ink. This inspired Hahnemann and five of his colleagues to do the first formal proving of **SEPIA.**

From the symptoms brought out in that first proving, Hahnemann discovered the healing properties of **SEPIA,** which have been invaluable for probably millions of women over the last 250 years.

Women needing **SEPIA,** especially at the time of menopause, often have a long-standing history of hormonal imbalance. The story of one of my patients, whom I will call Claudia, demonstrates the classic presentation when the Vital Force needs **SEPIA.**

Claudia's menses started when she was 11 and from the very beginning she was miserable every time she had her period. She had severe menstrual cramps and would bleed so heavily that she often missed school for the first day or two of every cycle.

At age 12 her pediatrician prescribed birth control pills for her, which she took for 15 years. When she stopped taking them to get pregnant, the cramps and bleeding came back just like in "the bad old days," as she put it. However, instead of her periods coming monthly as they had when she was younger, they were now irregular and she and her husband, Daniel, had difficulty conceiving.

Eventually she and Daniel had a baby girl after several rounds of in vitro fertilization (IVF). Claudia didn't tolerate the fertility drugs very well but she persevered until she got pregnant. When I asked her about the pregnancy, she told me that "it was very rough." She'd had morning sickness almost every day for the first 4 months and her baby was 2 weeks overdue so she had her labor induced with Pitocin. The birth was difficult because her daughter Christina weighed almost nine pounds. As often happens during the birth of large babies, Claudia suffered a vaginal laceration and lost so much blood that she needed a blood transfusion.

Claudia had postpartum depression that lasted about 4 months. She stopped breastfeeding Christina when she was prescribed antidepressant medication, which she took for almost 2 years. Her menstrual periods were even worse than before the pregnancy and so she started back on the birth control pills.

Claudia and Daniel had planned to have more children. But Claudia was exhausted and couldn't bear the thought of another pregnancy, especially if it meant she would need to go through IVF again. After much discussion, they decided they were happy with one healthy daughter and Daniel underwent a vasectomy.

I met Claudia when she was 48 and she came to see me for a second opinion about whether she should have a hysterectomy (surgical removal of the uterus.) She told me that despite Daniel's vasectomy, she had stayed on birth control pills because every time she would try to stop them, the cramps and heavy bleeding returned and she would become anemic. She complained that she had not been able to lose weight, which she attributed to being on the pill for so many years.

In an attempt to stop the birth control pills, three years previously she underwent an endometrial ablation where the lining of the uterus is essentially destroyed to try to lessen or stop heavy menstrual flow. Unfortunately for Claudia, it didn't work. She still had irregular, heavy bleeding and the cramps were so painful she had to take pain medication during every period. So, her doctor put her back on a low-dose birth control pill.

We calculated that she had been on some kind of hormonal therapy, either birth control pills or fertility drugs, for 35 of her 48 years. This may sound extreme, but it's not uncommon. In my experience, for most women with a history of menstrual problems starting at puberty, this is the norm.

Besides painful, heavy menses and a weight gain of 20 pounds that she could not lose despite years of yo-yo dieting and valiant attempts to exercise (which she hated to do), Claudia told me that she and Daniel's marriage was in trouble. Part of the problem was that she had absolutely no sex drive. Although she loved Daniel, she would cringe when he touched her and she didn't know why.

She complained of a feeling of pressure in her pelvis that was always worse after intercourse. She would go to great lengths to avoid having sex because of the pain. This put a great strain on her relationship with Daniel because the more he voiced his frustration, the more irritated and cranky she became. She was so tired that at the end of the day she just wanted to sleep. Claudia told me she was afraid that Daniel would leave her if their sex life didn't improve.

Needless to say, Claudia cried during most of our consultation. She had been told that her only option was to have a hysterectomy if she wanted to be able to get off the pill. But Claudia was scared to death of hospitals and the thought of going under the knife terrified her. She had heard me talking about alternatives to hysterectomy during a radio interview and she was hopeful that I could help her.

Claudia and I had a discussion about her options and I recommended that she consider homeopathic treatment. I explained to her that hysterectomy was always an option for her but that it was a permanent one and could have unforeseen consequences. Over the years, I have treated many patients like Claudia who opted for hysterectomy. When they would return for their follow-up consultations 6 to 12 months after hysterectomy, many of them told me the same thing. Although they appreciated not having periods anymore, they now had other complaints. Many told me they had not felt well since their surgery; fatigue, weight gain, lost sex drive, and sometimes depression were common complaints.

I never understood why this was so common until I studied homeopathy. When the uterus and/or the ovaries are surgically removed, the Vital Force takes a big hit and becomes depleted. The greater the depletion, the more numerous and complex the symptoms it produces. Chinese medicine practitioners say that removing an organ leaves a hole in the chi field. Once I understood this, I tried everything I could to avoid removing a woman's uterus and ovaries unless there was cancer. This was a very difficult decision for me to make because I always loved doing surgery and I had developed a high level of skill and expertise after 30 years of training and clinical practice.

But I remembered the first premise of medicine, which is *primum non nocere*: first, do no harm. As my homeopathic skills increased, I have been able to offer my patients a less harmful form of therapy that gets at the cause of their illness and, in the vast majority of cases, lets them keep all their parts.

I discussed all this with Claudia and gave her a copy of my book to read that explains in detail how homeopathy works and what she could expect from homeopathic treatment. She thanked me and we agreed that she would read the book, talk it over with Daniel, and decide how she wanted to proceed.

Claudia and Daniel both read the book and returned for a homeopathic consultation. After a short talk with Daniel, Claudia and I spent about an hour together and she filled me in with more details of her life's story. The remedy I recommended for her was **SEPIA;** her life story, all her symptoms, and the effects of prolonged hormone therapy and the endometrial ablation were a textbook case indicating **SEPIA** was the remedy she needed.

Because she was so depleted, I had her start with a daily dose of the lowest potency, the 6c. I changed her hormone therapy to bioidentical progesterone for 2 weeks of each month rather than have her stop the birth control pills cold turkey. I advised her to take the remedy *after* she took the progesterone; the remedy doesn't interfere with the action of the hormones but the hormones energetically interfere with the action of the remedy.

I saw Claudia 6 weeks later and she told me she was sleeping a little better. She had had one period and the bleeding wasn't quite as heavy. Her sex drive was still low, however—as it had been all her adult life.

I reassured her that this was good progress and we increased the potency of the remedy to the 9c. When she returned 6 weeks later, she reported that she felt less irritable and her mood was lighter. Claudia continued to take the remedy in increasing potency and have regular follow-up consultations with me. Her menstrual flow continued to get lighter, and after 6 months, she was able to stop the progesterone. For the first time since age 12, except when she was pregnant, she was taking no hormone therapy. Her sex drive gradually increased and the feeling of pressure in her pelvis went away after about 18 months. Claudia and Daniel have a healthy sex life and they both report that Claudia is less irritable and overall much happier.

It has been 6 years since Claudia started homeopathic treatment and she continues to take **SEPIA.** She is currently taking a very high potency and she needs the remedy adjusted about every 3 months. When it's time to adjust the potency, she complains of that heavy feeling in her pelvis again and she usually feels more irritable. She told me sometimes Daniel will ask her if she's due to have her remedy adjusted because he notices the difference in her mood.

Three years ago, she went through menopause and had her last period ("Hallelujah!" she said). Taking **SEPIA** helped her manage the hot flashes and night sweats; sometimes just taking an extra dose of the remedy was enough to do the trick.

During our most recent consultation, we talked about how much longer Claudia will need treatment. She told me that she has never felt this good in her entire life. She managed to lose about 10 pounds and she is happy with that. She has a lot of energy and sleeps like a baby most nights.

I told her I didn't know how much longer she would need the remedy but we discussed what signs to watch for that would tell us she is finished with **SEPIA.** If she is like most people, some of her initial symptoms like irritability and that heavy feeling in the pelvis will most likely return. We'll increase the potency but if her symptoms worsen or don't go away, I'll have her stop the remedy and see what happens. If her Vital Force no longer needs **SEPIA,** it will let us know by removing all her symptoms once she stops the remedy. As in the initial proving of **SEPIA**, she is now a healthy person and taking the remedy brings on the symptoms rather than relieving them. Whether or not she will need another, different remedy remains to be seen. But for now, she feels very well and she still has all her parts.

PMS/MENSTRUAL CRAMPS

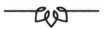

Just as there are homeopathic remedies to help women during menopause, of course there are remedies to help with other female complaints such as premenstrual syndrome (PMS), abnormal menstrual bleeding patterns, and painful periods. Before we discuss the remedies that are available to help with these issues, my training and years of practice as an obstetrician and gynecologist dictate that I say a word or two about when you can take care of yourself with over-the-counter remedies and when you should seek the help of a health practitioner.

Going through puberty and having monthly menstrual periods, by definition, turns us from girls into women. In many cultures, this is honored and celebrated as a rite of passage. I remember Dr. Christiane Northrup, author of *Women's Bodies, Women's Wisdom*, talking about marking the specialness of the day when her daughters started their periods. I don't recall all the details but what imprinted it on my memory was the fact that these were special life events that were acknowledged in their family.

Unfortunately, in our culture we tend to medicalize this normal part of the female life cycle. Over the years, I have had to reassure countless mothers that their daughters don't need a pelvic exam as soon as they start having periods. Menarche, or the onset of periods, is unique to each girl as she becomes a woman. It's not uncommon for her periods to be irregular at first; over time, they become regular in the vast majority of cases.

But, sometimes, as we saw in the case of Claudia, women can struggle with hormonal problems and menstrual troubles from the very beginning. In conventional medicine, the tools your doctor has to offer when things don't go smoothly are actually pretty few. As doctors, we're trained to treat symptoms and we do this by either prescribing pharmaceutical drugs or performing surgery. Homeopathy offers an alternative that gets at the underlying cause rather than just suppressing the symptoms. In each unique case, there is something that has upset the balance and harmony of the Vital Force.

There are myriad reasons why girls and women suffer from PMS, abnormal bleeding, menstrual cramps, and complications during pregnancy. Dr. Samuel Hahnemann understood that anything that disrupts the healthful economy of any living being does so by assaulting the Vital Force. He called such an assault a morbific influence inimical to life. This is why homeopaths are so concerned about learning the details of and the circumstances surrounding a particular illness or malady. It is in the **story** the patient tells that the homeopath seeks to uncover this inimical influence and choose the right remedy that resonates with the weakened Vital Force and can be used to restore it vibrationally to its normal, powerful state of well-being.

In this way, there is no *one* remedy that will work to relieve PMS or relieve menstrual pain, for example, in every woman. Each woman's life story is unique and the circumstances of her life reveal what is needed to the practitioner who is trained to listen to the language of the Vital Force.

So how do you know when you can try over-the-counter remedies to help yourself or your daughters and when you should consult your doctor? PMS and menstrual cramps are annoying and can be sometimes debilitating in extreme cases. However, they are not life threatening (unless there are guns in the house, just kidding!). Paying attention to how you feel or listening closely to your daughter when she's suffering can help you choose one of the few dozen remedies available over the counter that can help.

Understanding a little about the circumstances that attend the onset of the trouble, along with matching the symptoms, will help you make the best calculation on which remedy to try first. If you don't notice any relief after several doses of the first remedy, try another that looks close. In the end, you have nothing to lose by trying and you will learn a lot in the process. The worst thing that can happen in cases of menstrual cramps or PMS is that you resort to over-the-counter medications or prescription drugs in severe cases. These conditions are short lived and eventually the symptoms go away as the cycle progresses. If they persist despite your best efforts to choose a remedy, it's time to consult a homeopath.

However, when it comes to heavy or very irregular bleeding that occurs out of nowhere and lasts for more than one or two cycles, I advise that you see a conventional health practitioner trained in caring for women. This is especially true in cases of postmenopausal bleeding. Abnormal bleeding can be a sign of more serious conditions such as uterine or cervical cancer and should never be ignored. During pregnancy, any bleeding requires immediate consultation with your obstetrician or midwife.

If your health care practitioner confirms that there is nothing seriously wrong, I would advise seeing a homeopathic practitioner to recommend a remedy to help correct the imbalance in the Vital Force that is wreaking havoc with your menstrual cycle. There are more than 350 remedies that have abnormal menstrual bleeding as part of their symptom picture. It is almost impossible to choose the correct remedy solely on one symptom of heavy menses. Fewer than 25 of these remedies are available over the counter and the differences in their symptom picture can be very subtle. A deeper understanding of the nature of each remedy is often needed when trying to restore harmony to the hormonal system.

So, with these caveats duly noted, let's learn about some of the remedies that hold a special place in my heart and in my practice for the relief they offer girls and women at all stages of the life cycle.

We've already met the first remedy when we covered remedies for anxiety, asthma, colds, and headaches. **ACONITUM NAPELLUS**, called **ACONITE** for short, can be helpful in cases of **PMS**, where there is an intense **aggravation of the emotions** when the period starts. The *Materia Medica* describes this as "**frenzy or fury on the appearance of bleeding**." As we discussed previously, the energy of **ACONITE** is one of **suddenness, intensity**, and **anxiety** or **outright fear.**

I once used this remedy for a young woman who developed a severe case of PMS shortly after she was injured in a serious motor vehicle accident. Prior to the accident, her menstrual cycle was normal and she had no symptoms during her period. After the **shock** of being seriously injured, she became **very agitated and angry** when her period started. She was quite **anxious** and **couldn't sleep** for the first 2 days of bleeding. She developed **severe menstrual cramps** that would cause her to double over and her **flow was much heavier** than before the accident.

Her mother brought her to see me after her family doctor prescribed Xanax for her to take on the first day of her cycle to calm her down. As an alternative, I recommended **ACONITE** daily in a low potency. Over the next several months, we gradually increased the potency and within about 8 months her periods returned to their normal pattern, the PMS went away, and she was able to stop the **ACONITE**. The remedy succeeded in removing the energetic imprint on her Vital Force that occurred at the time of the accident.

ANTIMONIUM CRUDUM, the remedy discussed in the section on indigestion, is another helpful remedy for **PMS**, especially if **nausea** is part of the picture. This remedy also has the unique symptom of **toothache before the period starts.** It's also very helpful for *vomiting and diarrhea in pregnancy that persists past the first trimester.*

Water retention can be an annoying and sometimes uncomfortable **PMS** symptom for some women. **APIS MELLIFICA**, one of our best remedies for **swelling** of any kind, can relieve puffiness in the hands and feet that often occurs at the onset of menses. It's also helpful for **menstrual pain**, particularly when the pain feels like it's coming from the **ovaries.**

The miracles of **ARNICA MONTANA** are covered in more detail in the section on trauma, but it is worth mentioning here for the friend it can be to women in painful circumstances. **ARNICA** is the first remedy to use in **injuries of any kind** and thus it can work miracles in cases of **injury to the vagina from rape, childbirth, or overzealous intercourse**.

I once took care of a young girl who developed a massive hematoma (blood clot) from a **straddle injury** caused by falling into a swimming pool. Although it required surgery to evacuate the clot from the vulva and tie off the torn artery, giving her **ARNICA** 30c every few hours before and after surgery prevented the massive bruising that usually accompanies such an injury. It also decreased the amount of pain medication she needed postoperatively.

Lastly, this remedy is invaluable for pregnant women who develop **spotting or bleeding** due to a **threatened miscarriage after a fall or an accident.** Giving **ARNICA** 30c immediately and frequently on the way to the obstetrician's office or the hospital may save the pregnancy. Homeopathic remedies are safe to give during pregnancy at any stage when the proper remedy is chosen.

When we were teenagers, my sister Betsy and I had horrible cramps for the first day of our periods. As often happens with women living in the same home, we cycled at the same time and once a month we'd be confined to bed. I'll never forget the tongue lashing our mother gave our doctor when he told her, in front of us, that it was all in our heads and we were just trying to get out of going to school once a month! The only thing that seemed to help was a heating pad and large amounts of Pamprin®. If only I knew then what I know now. The remedy we needed was **ARSENICUM ALBUM**.

Like the name implies, it's made homeopathically from arsenic and, like its source, one of its keynote symptoms is ***severe cramping***. You'll recall ***cramping in the gut*** is part of the symptom picture of ***food poisoning*** when **ARSENICUM** is needed. **ARSENICUM** is one of those chilly remedies and menstrual pain asking for **ARSENICUM** is ***ameliorated by the application of heat***. If you crave a heating pad or hot water bottle on your belly during your period, taking **ARSENICUM** is a good alternative to ibuprofen or acetaminophen.

BELLADONNA is the remedy to consider for menstrual cramps when the ***blood is bright red, hot,*** and ***comes out in a gush.*** This remedy has helped many of my patients who complain the bleeding is so heavy that they can't get up off the toilet long enough to get a pad or a tampon. This remedy is also helpful for ***afterpains*** in postpartum mothers where there is ***cutting pain*** in the uterus when the baby nurses.

The section on growing pains discusses **CALCAREA PHOSPHORICA.** Just as it is helpful for headaches in school-aged children, it's also helpful for girls with late onset of their first period. For young women who ***bleed every 2 weeks*** or ***spot in between*** their monthly cycles, **CALC PHOS** can help to regulate the cycle when given daily over time. Remember this is a remedy for people who **crave smoked meat**. So, if your daughter begs for bacon every time her period is about to start, this is probably her remedy. **Menstrual cramps and severe backache** are also common symptoms indicating the need for **CALC PHOS.**

CAULLOPHYLLUM, made from the plant blue cohosh, is a remedy that is a true blessing for women. It's very helpful for women who have **severe cramps when there is very little menstrual flow,** usually at the onset of the period. But its greatest gift is to pregnant women about to go into labor. This remedy has been a crucial part of the birthing kit for homeopathic midwives for centuries. It has the ability to strengthen the Vital Force to harmonize sporadic uterine contractions in cases of false labor where the muscle fibers of the uterus are not firing together. **CAULLOPHYLLUM** helps to synchronize the uterine contractions to more effectively dilate the cervical opening to allow the baby to pass into the birth canal.

The next remedy has a very peculiar symptom that I have heard reported from only a very few patients over the years. **CAUSTICUM** patients report that their **menstrual flow stops during the night** while they sleep but starts up again in the morning. When they suffer from PMS, a **depressed mood** and a **feeling of weakness** can be part of the picture. Women needing **CAUSTICUM** often have another distinct characteristic in that they **cannot support injustice.** They feel badly when they see others treated unfairly and are usually quick to take up a cause or rally to the side of the underdog.

Just like the relief it brings for **irritable, teething babies,** **CHAMOMILLA** is the remedy to think of when **menstrual pain presents with extreme irritability or anger.** I still remember the first time I saw a woman in labor cursing out her husband every time she would have a contraction. The harder the contraction, the more she would scream—not only at her poor husband but at every one of us who tried to help her. Once the baby was delivered, she was perfectly calm and apologized profusely to everyone in the room.

This was many years before I had even heard about homeopathy but I realize now how many laboring women (and their husbands) could have benefitted if I had known then of the soothing power of **CHAMOMILLA.**

As the baby grows inside its mother's womb, it is surrounded by her energy field or what the Chinese call **chi.** So, it's not unusual that a baby will often need the same remedy that its mother needs. We know that **CHAMOMILLA** is a very effective remedy for **colic** where the baby is intensely irritable, even angry. So, it would not be uncommon for the baby of a mother needing **CHAMOMILLA** during labor to develop colic because the baby also needs **CHAMOMILLA.** This is why homeopaths ask about the mother's pregnancy and labor when they are treating an infant; determining what remedy the mother needs is very often the clue to the remedy that will bring her baby relief.

Women needing **CHAMOMILLA** seem to be especially **aggravated by drinking coffee**. In my experience, these women should avoid it because it often stops the action of the remedy and makes them feel even more irritated.

In the section on diarrhea, we encountered the remedy **CHINA OFFICIANALIS.** One of the distinct features of this remedy is ailments brought on by the **loss of vital fluids.** So, it should come as no surprise that **CHINA** is one of our most helpful remedies for women who suffer from very **heavy menstrual bleeding**. One of the most distinct symptoms in women who need this remedy is a **feeling of being totally wiped out** every time they have a menstrual cycle. This feeling can come before, during, or after the onset of bleeding but, in my experience, most women needing **CHINA** feel exhausted for at least a week to 10 days every month.

Giving **CHINA** daily as a constitutional remedy has brought vitality back for many women who have long suffered from years of heavy bleeding and literally feel completely drained. If you think this is the remedy you need, taking it only during the menses is often not enough to permanently restore your Vital Force. Taking it daily in ever-increasing potencies over time is usually necessary to completely relieve the **weakness** and **fatigue**. A consultation with a homeopath can give you the information you need on how often to take the remedy and when it is time to stop it.

The next remedy helpful for women during the menses is **CIMICIFUGA RACEMOSA**, made from the plant black cohosh. Whereas its cousin **CAULLOPHYLLUM**, the homeopathic preparation of blue cohosh, is particularly helpful for women in the early stages of labor, the action of **CIMICIFUGA** is more suited to women with **pain that increases with the amount of menstrual flow.** There are some peculiar symptoms that are clues to the use of this remedy. The first is the aggravation caused by becoming cold. **Menstrual pain that is worse in cold weather** or after being exposed to cold calls for **CIMICIFUGA**.

In addition, there is often **pain in the joints** or the **upper back** during menses when **CIMICIFUGA** is needed. Women needing this remedy will often complain of feeling like they have a black cloud that hangs over them while they are bleeding but lifts once their period is over.

I once used this remedy for a woman who had severe arthritis pain that would come on only during her period which was very heavy. Once she had a hysterectomy to stop the heavy bleeding, the arthritis pain occurred daily. In homeopathy, we call this **ailments from suppressed menses.** Removing the uterus stops the flow of blood but it doesn't restore the imbalance in the Vital Force. In fact, it often weakens the Vital Force and that is why this patient's arthritis pain got worse after her hysterectomy.

By the time I saw her in consultation, she had been suffering with arthritis pain in her back, hands, and feet for more than 10 years. She was also very depressed and didn't like having to take antidepressants as well as pain medication. Once she started on **CIMICIFUGA**, first in low potency, then in increasingly higher potencies, her mood lifted and her back pain completely resolved. Over time, the arthritis pain in her hands and feet also went away and she was able to stop both the pain medications and the antidepressant.

As we saw with the remedy **CHINA**, **COCCULUS INDICUS** is another remedy for women who complain of feeling **weak** and **fatigued** every time their period starts. While CHINA is the remedy for women who become wiped out from heavy bleeding, the exhaustion of **COCCULUS** is usually precipitated by taking care of sick children or an ailing parent. Remember this is the remedy to consider for **ailments from night watching**, or **nursing the sick.**

The weakness that comes on during menses is sometimes so severe, the **COCCULUS** patient can barely get out of bed. They often have *menstrual cramps* with a feeling of *swelling or distention in the uterus* as well.

Just as **COLOCYNTHIS** is helpful for relieving abdominal cramping, it is a remedy to try for *menstrual cramps that are better bending over double.* Women needing **COLOCYNTHIS** during their period often get *relief by applying firm pressure*. I once had a patient who told me that what really helped her menstrual cramps was to have her cat lie on her belly.

CUPRUM METALLICUM, a remedy often given for leg cramps, can also help relieve *cramps* in the uterus *during menses.* It's another remedy that can help with the *cramping pain that persists in the uterus after childbirth*, especially in women who have had multiple pregnancies. The cramps can be quite severe and sometimes the pain radiates up into the chest. The *Materia Medica* indicates it is helpful for menstrual problems brought on by *suppressed foot sweat* but I admit I've never heard any woman complain of that. I'm not even sure how one stops their feet from sweating but homeopaths from past centuries repeatedly mention this peculiar symptom so I'm sure it has helped women in the past.

In the early days of my practice, I cared for a college student who was referred to me by her dermatologist for a very specific problem. Every time her period started, she would break out in a red, blotchy rash all over her torso. It always started the first day of her menses and she would always have menstrual cramps at the same time. After her period stopped, the rash and the pain went away until the next month. This was before I had studied homeopathy and I had little to offer her except birth control pills. Unfortunately, she couldn't tolerate the pill because it gave her headaches.

What I didn't know at the time is that the homeopathic remedy she needed was **DULCAMARA.** Like the remedy **CIMICIFUGA, DULCAMARA** patients are ***aggravated by cold weather***. The other peculiar presentation of this remedy is ***herpes outbreaks*** that return when the ***weather turns cold.***

GELSMEMIUM SEMPERVIRENS, the remedy that is so helpful for the ***flu***, also has a role to play in helping women who have ***dysmenorrhea*** (painful periods) with ***migraine*** and ***vomiting.*** Imagine having a migraine every time you start your period! Taking **GELSEMIUM** at the first sign of the migraine aura or the menstrual cramps can prevent a full-blown migraine from developing. As in most cases of migraine headaches, taking a remedy on a regular basis over time is usually needed to stop the cyclical pattern.

Do you remember the incident I mentioned about the surgical patients who developed postoperative bleeding due to a bad batch of suture? The remedy that helped them was **HAMAMELLIS VIRGINIANA,** made from witch hazel. This remedy has helped many of my patients who have had a history of ***very heavy, prolonged periods*** that often last more than a week. It's a wonderful remedy for women who spot or bleed in between periods as well.

HAMAMELLIS also has a rare and peculiar symptom called ***vicarious menstruation.*** No, this doesn't mean that someone else has your period for you! It means that instead of the normal menstrual flow, bleeding comes from other sites like the nose or even the rectum. In conventional medicine, we would attribute such a phenomenon to bleeding from endometriosis, a condition where the uterine lining, or endometrium, ends up in places where it doesn't belong. Because this tissue is under hormonal control, it bleeds during the onset of the menstrual period just as if it were located in its normal place inside the uterus. I once cared for a patient with severe endometriosis who would bleed from an endometrial implant in her navel whenever her period started. **PHOSPHORUS** is another remedy that has this unusual symptom as part of its symptom presentation.

BRYONIA, the remedy we learned about for any ***complaints that are worse from motion,*** also has ***vicarious menstruation***. Women needing **BRYONIA** can have ***nosebleeds with or instead of their regular menstrual flow.*** This is one of the many things I love about homeopathy. Even in the most bizarre or unusual cases, there truly is a remedy for everything!

Another common menstrual complaint is ***absent or missed*** periods, also known as ***amenorrhea.*** Of course, the most common reason for amenorrhea in reproductive-age women is pregnancy. There are about 300 homeopathic remedies that can be used to manage missed periods and this problem requires professional consultation.

Delayed menarche, or late onset of the first menses at the time of puberty, should also be treated by a professional homeopath. However, there is one available remedy that I have found to be very helpful for young girls whose ***period is often late to start*** and when it does, there is often ***severe pain and cramping***. This remedy is **PULSATILLA NIGRICANS. *Nervousness and/or tearfulness*** is not uncommon in young women who need **PULSATILLA**. As with young children who need this remedy for ***fever due to ear infections***, ***weeping*** and ***a desire to be comforted*** are prominent symptoms.

SABINA is a remedy that is well suited for women with ***heavy periods*** where the ***blood is bright red and mixed with dark clots.*** The ***menstrual pain that is better*** when ***lying on the back*** is a clue to **SABINA**. The pain often radiates from the small of the back through the pelvis to the pubic bone, and as in the remedy **BRYONIA**, the pain is *worse with the slightest motion*. Women often complain of *pain shooting up into the vagina* when this remedy is needed.

As discussed at length in the section on menopause, **SEPIA SUCCUS** is one of the most important remedies for women. *Irregular menses*, with either a *light or a heavy flow,* can be helped by taking **SEPIA** if all the other symptoms fit the picture. **SEPIA,** as well as several other remedies, including **CIMICIFUGA,** can be used to help women with *prolapse of the uterus*. A sense of *heaviness in the pelvis*, like my patient Claudia had, or the ability to actually feel the uterus in the lower part of the vagina are the most usual symptoms consistent with uterine prolapse. On pelvic examination, it is clear that the uterus is not in its normal location high in the vaginal canal and there is actually a grading system used to describe the degree of prolapse.

James Tyler Kent, MD, was one of the most prominent practitioners and professors of homeopathy in America at the end of the 19th century. His *Lectures on Homeopathic Materia Medica* has been a standard textbook for students of homeopathy since its publication in 1905 and it is still used to this day. From his lecture on **CIMICIFUGA,** I learned something that would have been dismissed as impossible by my gynecology professors. *"It is true that remedies will cure prolapsus when the symptoms agree, and at no other time. If it fits the patient in general, these bearing down sensations will go away, the patient will be made comfortable, and an examination will finally show that the parts are in normal condition.* ***You cannot prescribe for the prolapsus; you must prescribe for the woman.***

You cannot prescribe for one symptom, because there are probably 50 remedies that have that symptom."

Once my skills as a homeopath increased, I found this to be true and I continue to recommend homeopathic remedies for my patients with varying degrees of uterine prolapse. Except in extreme cases where the entire uterus is protruding from the vagina, homeopathy has brought relief to many of my patients with uterine prolapse when the remedy fits the patient in general. I have found homeopathy particularly helpful in older women who suffer from uterine prolapse and are not good surgical candidates. In many cases, I have found that a well-chosen homeopathic remedy in combination with a pessary, a mechanical device that supports the uterus in place, is sufficient to bring women relief and help them to avoid surgery.

In addition to **ARNICA MONTANA**, the trauma remedy, there is another remedy that is invaluable for women who have survived *rape or sexual abuse.* That remedy is **STAPHYSAGRIA**, which is made from the seeds of the delphinium flower. In addition to being one of the primary remedies for *urinary tract infections*, **STAPHYSAGRIA** is also a remedy for *uterine prolapse* and for *pain after intercourse,* especially in virgins. It is also a remedy for vaginal warts caused by the human papilloma virus, *when all the patient's symptoms fit the profile of STAPHYSAGRIA.* The *Materia Medica* lists this remedy as useful for amenorrhea from indignation, but I must admit I've never had a patient recount such a history to me. Unlike **SEPIA**, **STAPHYSAGRIA** often has a very high sex drive that can even border on what the early homeopaths called nymphomania. *Unsatisfied sexual desire in widows* is another **STAPHYSAGRIA** symptom mentioned repeatedly in many of the textbooks from the 19th century.

Like the prominent headache remedy, **NATRUM MURIATICUM, SULPHUR** is one of the over-the-counter remedies to consider when *headaches start just before the menstrual period.* The skin is one of the primary areas where **SULPHUR** manifests many symptoms and it often brings relief to women who complain of *itching of the vulva. Excessive sweating of the genitals with a strong odor* is also a common symptom relieved by taking homeopathic **SULPHUR.** This is a common symptom that most women only discuss with their gynecologist and there are other remedies that have this symptom also. However, the two over-the-counter remedies to try for this annoying complaint are **SULPHUR** and **THUJA.**

THUJA is a remedy like **STAPHYSAGRIA** that can be used to treat *venereal warts* caused by the *human papilloma virus,* or *HPV,* in both men and women. Once again, the characteristics of the remedy must fit the overall symptoms of the patient. Cases where *venereal warts* or *condylomata* have grown extensively over the outer genitals or involve the cervix usually require long-term homeopathic treatment and are best treated with the help of a professional homeopath. However, in cases where there are just one or two small warts, especially if they appear after receiving a vaccination, **THUJA** in the 30c potency daily may help. However, if the warts continue to grow or more of them erupt, this is a sign from the Vital Force that you either need a different remedy or a change in potency.

THUJA is also one of 85 remedies that is commonly used by professional homeopaths for *adverse reactions after vaccination.* The mental symptoms indicating **THUJA** tend toward *depression* and a *feeling of isolation.*

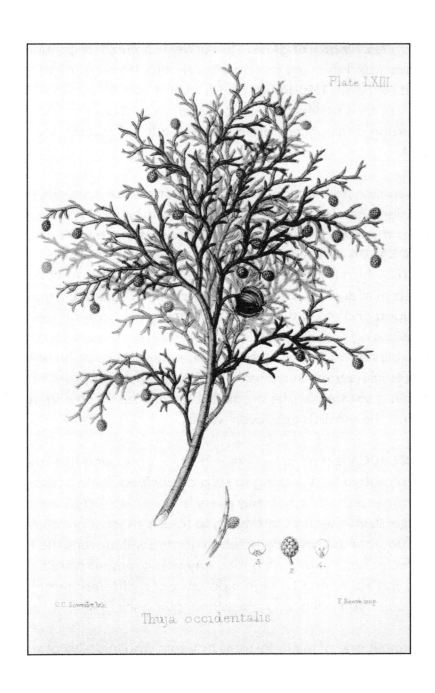

Plate LXIII.

C.C.Sowerby lith.   F.Reeve imp.

Thuja occidentalis.

1.   3.   2.   4.

131

One of the classic symptoms of this remedy is a feeling that they are *fragile or made of glass.* One of my patients is a gentleman who described this very feeling after he slipped on some black ice and hit his head. **THUJA** has had a remarkable effect on him and he relates that he feels stronger and more confident in himself, and his thinking and concentration have greatly improved since taking **THUJA.**

No discussion on homeopathic remedies that are a special help to women would be complete without mentioning **PHYTOLACCA.** Besides the indication for *sore throat radiating to the ears,* **PHYTOLACCA** is especially helpful for nursing mothers who develop *mastitis,* which is inflammation of the breast usually from a blocked milk duct. In conventional medicine, antibiotics are usually prescribed and often this leads to weaning the baby off the breast and switching to formula feedings. Mastitis presents with a hard, red, swollen mass in the breast that is exquisitely painful to the touch. Nursing from that breast becomes almost impossible because the pain is so intense. The breast then becomes more engorged with milk and the mastitis gets even worse.

PHYTOLACCA is a miracle worker in these cases and has saved many a mother from having to stop breastfeeding. In acute cases, I recommend the 30c potency every hour or two. Often the relief is almost instantaneous. Continuing to take it at least once or twice a day until the breast is completely normal will prevent the mastitis from recurring. If you don't notice *any* improvement after five or six doses, you either need a higher potency or a different remedy; in either case, you will need professional guidance.

Marianne is one of my long-term patients who initially consulted me for help with a long history of recurrent sinus infections and severe sensitivity to chemicals. She started on **MAGNESIUM CARBONICUM**, a constitutional remedy that fit all her symptoms. Gradually, her health improved and she became less chemically sensitive and could tolerate going places that she had previously avoided. Increasing the potency and frequency of her regular remedy or adding remedies when she got a sinus infection helped her to avoid taking multiple courses of antibiotics which had been her usual treatment since she was a child. Then, Marianne developed a severe case of mastitis of the left breast at age 61.

When she came to see me, she had a painful, tennis ball-sized red area on her left breast. It was so tender and swollen that she couldn't bear to have anything touch her skin, much less wear a bra. She had a fever of 100.9°F and a blood-tinged discharge from the nipple. The interesting thing about Marianne's case was that she had developed a case of mastitis in the exact same place on the same breast while she was nursing her son more than 35 years ago. Of course, at that time, she was given antibiotics and told to stop nursing.

Because Marianne had had good homeopathic treatment for years before this episode, this condition is the result of the constitutional remedy annihilating a disease that had been suppressed for 35 years. This is called *return of old symptoms.* When Marianne's mastitis returned, I gave her four hourly doses of **PHYTOLACCA** 30c, the remedy she needed 35 years ago. Her temperature dropped to 99.9°F with minor improvement in her level of pain. I increased her constitutional remedy, **MAGNESIUM CARBONICUM**, to LM34 daily and had her go up to **PHYTOLACCA** 200c every 2 hours through the night. The following day, she had no fever and felt considerably better, with less tenderness and considerably less redness.

She continued **PHYTOLACCA** 200c every hour and I had her order the next higher potency of **PHYTOLACCA**, 1M (1,000c), just in case it was needed. Because inflammatory breast cancer can present this way, I sent her for a breast MRI, which was suspicious for ductal carcinoma in situ, an early form of breast cancer. We increased the remedy to **PHYTOLACCA** 1M daily, and she got three opinions regarding the diagnosis. It was agreed that a biopsy was warranted and I concurred. The biopsy revealed a benign intraductal papilloma, a simple polyp.

She continued **PHYTOLACCA** 1M daily, the abscess slowly resolved, and the nipple discharge became clear yellow. After four months, all the breast symptoms resolved, and the **PHYTOLACCA** was stopped.

To this day, Marianne continues to take the same constitutional remedy and she is now on the LM260 potency of **MAGNESIUM CARBONICUM**. She has needed intercurrent remedies at times for other acute problems but her overall health has greatly improved from the sickliness she suffered as a child and young adult. Her latest mammogram this past August was completely normal.

MORNING SICKNESS

Nausea, with or without vomiting, or morning sickness, is not uncommon in the early stages of pregnancy and usually stops after about the third month. In severe cases, called hyperemesis gravidarum, there is such severe nausea with constant vomiting that the mother can become dehydrated. This requires medical attention and sometimes rehydration with intravenous fluids is necessary. But for garden variety nausea in pregnancy, there are several remedies available to you over the counter that can bring relief.

Here's what one of our wisest homeopaths, Dr. James Tyler Kent, had to say about treating morning sickness homeopathically. "Kali carb. is often a remedy for vomiting in pregnancy, but to find out when it is the remedy for vomiting of pregnancy, we have to go to the whole constitutional state. Vomiting of pregnancy is not cured, although it may be temporarily relieved, by ipecac, as this is a medicine that corresponds merely to the nausea itself... The condition really depends upon the constitutional state, and the remedy that is to cure must be a constitutional remedy. Sulphur, Sepia, and Kali carb. are among the remedies commonly indicated."

So, when you're trying to determine which remedy will relieve your morning sickness, paying close attention to all your symptoms as well as your mood and temperament can help you choose the correct remedy without too much trial and error. As always, if your attempts don't meet with success, consulting a homeopath who knows these remedies well can help.

It will come as no surprise that our mainstay remedy for **food poisoning**, **ARSENICUM ALBUM**, would also be very helpful for women whose sensitive stomachs become especially aggravated when they're pregnant. These women **cannot bear the sight or smell of food.** Anything they do manage to eat or drink comes right back up. Sometimes there can be retching or dry heaves even when the stomach is empty. In these cases, dehydration can come on fairly quickly. **Vomiting with diarrhea** is another common symptom indicating **ARSENICUM ALBUM**. When given in the 30c potency under the tongue, this remedy relieves the nausea and vomiting.

However, drinking very cold water will cause vomiting again. Women needing **ARSENICUM** prefer small sips of liquids instead of drinking large amounts at one time.

Remember, **ARSENICUM** is an *anxious* remedy and when women needing this remedy are sick, they often worry that something is terribly wrong. **ARSENICUM** patients worry about their health and the health of the ones they love. So, if you notice that you are more anxious than usual when the nausea strikes, **ARSENICUM** would be the first remedy to try.

COCCULUS INDICUS is another remedy that helps relieve *morning sickness*, especially for women who are prone to *motion sickness.* This remedy is often indicated for mothers of small children who become pregnant and have severe morning sickness. You'll recall that **COCCULUS** is one of the remedies for *ailments from night watching* or *nursing the sick*. So, it stands to reason that mothers who may become worn out from caring for their sick toddler will develop nausea during pregnancy because the Vital Force is asking for the restorative help of **COCCULUS**. Taking this remedy relieves the *morning sickness* as well as the *fatigue*.
As we shall see later, **COCCULUS** is a must-have remedy for travelers because of its great ability to prevent or relieve *motion sickness.*

I once cared for a pregnant woman who confessed to me that her morning sickness was so bad, she had to sleep with a bucket beside her bed. The moment she woke up and turned over in bed, she would vomit. The remedy she needed was **CUPRUM METALLICUM.** The morning sickness of **CUPRUM** comes on *first thing in the morning* and is *aggravated by the slightest motion*. Just as **CUPRUM** can relieve *menstrual cramps*, it can also bring relief for *cramps* in the belly that occur *with morning sickness*. A case of the

hiccups that triggers a bout of vomiting is another indication the mother needs **CUPRUM.**

For some women, their **digestion slows during pregnancy** and they will actually **vomit undigested food** first thing in the morning before they eat breakfast. The remedy indicated for this awful symptom is **FERRUM PHOSPHORICUM**, one of our best **cold remedies. Severe nausea that comes on suddenly** is another call for this remedy. **Stomach pain that gets worse after eating** is also helped by **FERRUM PHOS.**

Morning sickness that is triggered by the smell of cigarette smoke is a classic sign that the needed remedy is **IGNATIA AMARA.** This remedy is also very helpful for an odd condition we occasionally see in pregnant woman called **pica.**

Pica is condition where there is **a desire to eat indigestible things** such as dirt, paint, or starch. Women who get relief from eating nonnutritive things like this often need **IGNATIA.** In milder cases of pica, craving for ice is common and that's a feature of another remedy, **PHOSPHORUS.**

Most pregnant women with pica are embarrassed to admit they have such strange cravings but it's important to share this information with your obstetrician or midwife. Anemia is common in pregnant women with pica. A simple blood test can detect this. Treating the anemia will often resolve the desire to eat weird things. But if the cravings persist, especially in **pregnant women who are anxious or depressed**, **IGNATIA** is most likely the remedy needed.

Severe nausea that doesn't get better after vomiting is an indication for **IPECACAUNHA**. This remedy is made from the ipecac root, the source of syrup of ipecac, which can be used to induce vomiting in certain types of poisoning. Like **ARSENICUM, IPECACAUNHA** is a remedy for both *food poisoning* and *morning sickness*. But unlike the **ARSENICUM** patient, a mother needing **IPECACUAHNA** gets no relief from the nausea, no matter how many times she vomits. Constant retching and vomiting with dry heaving is a call for **IPECACUANHA.**

IPECACUANHA can also bring relief to *infants who vomit whenever they breastfeed.* Dissolve one pellet of the remedy in water and give a small amount to the baby if he or she vomits after nursing. A few doses of **IPECACUANHA** in a *vomiting infant* can promote breastfeeding which is healthier for babies than infant formula.

KALI CARBONICUM is another over-the-counter remedy that can relieve morning sickness especially in women with the other keynote symptoms of this remedy. *Weakness, intolerance to cold, sweating,* and *backache* are all hallmark symptoms of **KALI CARBONICUM.** Homeopathic midwives find this remedy especially helpful for women with back labor where all the pain is felt in the lower back instead of in the uterus.

Back labor is usually an indication that the baby is in a position called occiput posterior where the baby is coming through the pelvis face up instead of face down. I have seen cases like this where a properly given remedy actually helps the baby to turn during labor without any manipulation by the attendant. Obviously, this is not something to try at home but I mention it as one more testimony to the power of the correct homeopathic remedy to stimulate the Vital Force which then directs the action necessary to restore health or relieve suffering.

Pregnant women who suffer with morning sickness who *frequently vomit watery phlegm* often need **NATRUM MURIATICUM**. In cases where pregnant women are *nauseated and thirsty,* this is the remedy to consider. *Heartburn and belching after eating* are common in women needing **NAT MUR**.

PODOPHYLLUM is another over-the-counter remedy that is helpful for morning sickness. Like **FERRUM PHOSPORICUM, PODOPHYLLUM** patients have *weak digestion*. But instead of vomiting undigested food, the pregnant woman who needs *PODOPHYLLUM vomits mostly mucus* but has *burps that smell like rotten eggs*. Their *stomach is so weak* that they can barely digest simple foods like rice cereal and *heartburn with gagging* is often a problem.

Like **IPECACUANHA, PODOPHYLLUM** can be used to help *nursing infants who vomit after feeding*. But unlike **IPECACUANHA**, which works primarily on the stomach, **PODOPHYLLUM** also has action in the lower GI tract. Babies who need **PODOPHYLLUM** often have *profuse* amounts of *yellow or green diarrhea* that runs right through the diaper. What a relief this remedy is for parents of babies who leak at both ends! Remember to always place the pellet in water when giving a remedy to an infant to avoid the rare risk of choking. Infants and small children can often get by with just a few doses of the 6c potency.

Of course, **SEPIA SUCCUSS,** the premier women's remedy relieves morning sickness when the entire symptom picture fits. **SEPIA** has almost every variation of morning sickness including those *rotten egg belchings* seen with **PODOPHYLLUM**. *Nausea in the morning before eating*, and *nausea at the mere thought or smell of food*, as with **ARSENICUM**, are common in women needing **SEPIA**.

Frequent **vomiting after eating** or **vomiting up milky fluid** are also part of the symptom picture with **SEPIA**.

So, when a remedy like **SEPIA** has so many morning sickness symptoms in common with other remedies, how do you know which remedy to try first? Following the advice of Dr. Kent, matching all the symptoms with your constitution is needed to relieve all your symptoms, not just the nausea.

Recalling what we learned about **SEPIA** in the section on menopausal hot flashes, women who need **SEPIA** often have a history of "female trouble" from a young age. Women who have been on birth control pills for many years before they become pregnant are often in a **SEPIA** state. They tend to be **irritable** and their **sex drive** that was low before virtually disappears during pregnancy. In fact, **aversion to being touched by her husband** even though she loves him dearly is one of the hallmark symptoms of **SEPIA**.

Along with **KALI CARB** and **SEPIA**, **SULPHUR** is one of the three remedies Kent mentions in his *Lectures on Homeopathic Materia Medica* that are often indicated in cases of morning sickness. Like **FERRUM PHOSPHORICUM** and **PODOPHYLLUM**, pregnant women needing **SULPHUR** may **vomit undigested food** in the morning. **SULPHUR** is usually a remedy for women with **morning sickness at the very earliest stage** of their pregnancy. **Hot flashes** and **morning sickness** that come on within the first month or two of pregnancy often indicate **SULPHUR**.

Much has been written in our textbooks about the constitution of **SULPHUR,** as it was one of the original remedies proved by the great Hahnemann himself. Women who need **SULPHUR** are not too particular about their appearance and they are perfectly content to wear the same pair of sweat pants day after day. ***Hunger with a feeling of weakness at 11 o'clock*** in the morning is a classic **SULPHUR** symptom. ***Skin rashes and eruptions*** are also common, as the skin is one of the primary spheres of action for **SULPHUR.** ***Drinking milk*** often brings on a ***sour taste in the mouth*** with lots of *sour* **burping** and **belching. SULPHUR** patients also tend to be ***very thirsty*** and seem to always carry a water bottle with them. When I am considering whether one of my patients needs **SULPHUR,** I always ask them if they wear socks to bed. If their answer is an emphatic "No!" then that's another clue that **SULPHUR** is the remedy they need. SULPHUR patients tend to be **aggravated by the heat of the bed** and they prefer to ***sleep with their feet uncovered.***

Like **IGNATIA AMARA, TABACUM** is a remedy for morning sickness that is made much ***worse from the smell of tobacco smoke.*** As its name implies, this remedy is made from the tobacco plant. **TABACUM** patients always feel better if they can get out into the ***fresh air.*** Women needing **TABACUM** don't suffer as much emotionally like the woman who needs **IGNATIA** does. Morning sickness that is so severe that ***riding in a car or being on a boat is impossible*** calls for **TABACUM**. This is often true in cases where **COCCULUS** is needed but there are some differences between these two remedies that can help you figure out which one you need if you suffer from both morning sickness *and* motion sickness. (A double dose of misery!)

Remember that **COCCULUS** patients often feel ***weak and tired***, especially if they have been up at night caring for a sick child. The nausea and vomiting of **COCCULUS** is ***worse from the cold*** so the desire for fresh air is not as strong for **COCCULUS** patients as it is for those needing **TABACUM.**

When nausea is accompanied by the ***need to spit*** frequently, think of **TABACUM**. The ***vomiting of TABACUM is especially violent*** and the slightest motion will set it off. Another peculiar feature of **TABACUM** is that the patient feels ***better by uncovering the abdomen.*** As discussed next, **TABACUM** and **COCCULUS** are two of the primary remedies for ***motion sickness.***

MOTION SICKNESS

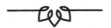

My parents tell me that when I was about 6 months old, I could not ride in a car, especially on winding roads, without vomiting during the entire trip. As a child, whenever we went on family trips, I always had to sit in the front seat; otherwise, I'd be sick to my stomach the entire time. This was actually a blessing in disguise as I wasn't crowded in the back seat of our Nash Rambler with my four other siblings!

After more than 25 years of using only homeopathic remedies to maintain and enhance my own health, I was recently surprised to find myself reading a book while riding in the back seat of a car without the customary nausea that had plagued me for years. This is something I had never been able to do in the past, especially when riding through the mountains of Colorado.

It illustrates for me, once again, the power of homeopathy to restore the Vital Force and remove symptoms that have been a part of our pattern for many years.

If I could go back in Professor Peabody's Wayback Machine (Google it, youngsters!), I would give my little girl self a dose of **TABACUM 30c** before any road trip. (Of course, then I would be stuck in the back seat with the rest of the brood!) Like most people in the 50s, our father was a heavy smoker and if he smoked while driving in the car, I would soon be heaving all over our poor mother. Getting out of the car and breathing some fresh air always made me feel better and that is the keynote symptom of **TABACUM.** (To his credit, the day the Surgeon General declared that cigarette smoking caused lung cancer, our father gave up a three-pack-a-day cigarette habit cold turkey. To this day, he is going strong at 86 and hasn't smoked a cigarette in over 50 years.)

In addition to relieving *morning sickness* like **TABACUM, COCCULUS INDICUS** is also one of our primary remedies for *motion sickness.* The motion sickness of **COCCULUS** often presents with a *headache* in addition to the nausea and vomiting. Like the remedy **BRYONIA**, the slightest motion aggravates the **COCCULUS** patient so much that even *moving their eyes* will make them feel *dizzy* and increase the *nausea.* This is why people needing **COCCULUS** not only feel sick when riding in a car or being on a boat, but just standing on the shore and *watching the movement of the boat can trigger a headache, nausea, and vomiting. Dizziness* and a *feeling they may faint* also plague the person needing **COCCULUS** as they reflect the weakened state that usually predisposes them to needing this remedy.

NUX VOMICA is another over-the-counter remedy that can be used for *motion sickness*. Remember this is the first remedy to think of in cases of a *hangover* where the body feels toxic from too much alcohol and/or rich food. *Indigestion, heartburn,* and *belching* are common **NUX** symptoms. All of these symptoms can be brought on by riding in a car or sailing on a ship in people who need **NUX.** The motion sickness of **TABACUM** or **COCCULUS** don't usually have the *heartburn*, *belching*, and *indigestion* we see when **NUX VOMICA** is indicated.

Taking this remedy can prevent the need to take antacids or pharmaceutical drugs called proton pump inhibitors that are often prescribed for GERD (gastroesophageal reflux disease).

PETROLEUM, or crude oil, was commonly used as a cure-all in the 19th and early 20th centuries. People would rub it on their skin for arthritis or after injuries. By applying the crude substance to the skin repeatedly, people essentially did a clinical proving on themselves. By observing patients who used the crude oil in this way, homeopaths were able to add symptoms to the *Materia Medica* that indicate when homeopathic **PETROLEUM** would bring relief.

Vertigo is part of the symptom picture in the motion sickness of **PETROLEUM**. The patient will feel as if the whole room is spinning. In addition to nausea and vomiting, headache involving the back of the head (occiput) is a common indication to give **PETROLEUM**.

Skin problems, especially *deep cracks in the fingers* that may bleed, are another feature pointing to homeopathic **PETROLEUM**. One of my clients diagnosed with colon cancer that had metastasized to the liver suffered with cracked fingers for years. **PETROLEUM** is one of the remedies he took as part of a regimen that helped him survive the side effects of chemotherapy and multiple surgeries. The cracks in his fingers greatly improved and are no longer as painful. Whenever his fingers begin to crack again, it's a sign from his Vital Force that it is time to change the frequency or potency of his remedies. After adjustments are made, his fingers heal and he feels better. He has lived longer than the statistics predicted and his oncology nurse refers to him as their miracle man.

TRAUMA

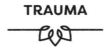

A number of years ago, I was making rounds in the hospital one morning when I encountered one of my colleagues, a geriatric specialist, who was making rounds with a group of medical residents. As we said our hellos, I could see he was in a lot of pain. He looked drawn and tired and he moved very gingerly. I asked him what was wrong and he told me this story.

A few months before, he had been climbing up Camelback Mountain in Phoenix and had strained his back. Ever since that day he had been suffering with **sciatica**, a shooting nerve pain that starts in the buttocks and runs down the leg.

He had tried physical therapy and even epidural injections of pain medications in his lower back to no avail. Although he would get some temporary relief after these therapies, the pain persisted. When I met him, he told me that his doctor had nothing else to offer him except narcotic pain meds, which is not an option for a doctor caring for very sick and dying patients. So, he was just trying to "white knuckle through it" and the toll it was taking on him was plainly evident on his face and in his cautious manner when he moved.

It seems like I had been a homeopath for about 20 minutes back in those days, but I recalled from Kent's *Repertory* there were only three remedies for sciatica after injury: **ARNICA, RUTA, and HYPERICUM.** I told my colleague that I might be able to help him. I went back to my office and put about 30 pellets of a remedy into a little envelope and dropped it off at his office with instructions on how to take it.

When I didn't hear back from him, I figured that he hadn't taken the remedy or, if he had, that I hadn't chosen correctly and he'd found no relief. But about a month later, I was back in the hospital and from down the hall I heard someone call out, "Kathi Fry, hypericum!" I turned around and the geriatrician was walking briskly without pain with a big grin on his face. He shook his leg and wiggled around a bit to show me that he was completely pain free.

He told me that he had taken the **HYPERICUM** 200c I had sent over three times a day and within a week he had no more pain. **HYPERICUM** is the *first remedy to consider for nerve pain* where there's that awful pins and needles feeling shooting down the limb. If my colleague had been my patient at the time of the injury, I would have advised him to take **ARNICA MONTANA** immediately as it is the *first remedy to take after injury* of any kind. Usually the 30c potency is sufficient but if the trauma is severe or the 30c doesn't seem to hold, use the 200c and repeat it every few hours. Taking **ARNICA** along with **HYPERICUM** at the time of the injury could have saved my colleague months of pain and expensive treatment.

Due to its propensity to relieve *nerve pain,* **HYPERICUM** is especially well suited to heal injuries to the most sensitive parts of the body that are rich in nerve endings such as the tips of the fingers or the toes. With **ARNICA, HYPERICUM** is the perfect remedy to give a baby **after circumcision**. Just place one pellet in water and give the baby a spoonful every hour or two until the pain subsides.

Nerve pain with tingling and numbness due to **dental work, spinal taps, whiplash,** or **injury to the tailbone** after a fall is almost miraculously relieved by the power of **HYPERICUM.** This remedy can also stop **muscle spasms** that occur after any injury. You can get the 30c potency in the health food store, but I recommend also having the 200c on hand in case the 30c doesn't bring lasting relief. (See resources for places to order remedies.)

The third remedy listed under **sciatica after injury**, is **RUTA GRAVEOLENS.** You may recall this remedy from the section on headaches, because it is a great remedy for **eye strain**. **RUTA** has a special affinity for the connective tissues, especially the flexor tendons when they become strained from **overuse**. **Tennis elbow** or **strained biceps tendons** in weightlifters are prime subjects for the healing power of **RUTA**. **Eye strain** occurs when overuse strains the small muscles, which are mostly tendinous, that move the eyeball. **Sciatic pain** caused by **injury to the fibrous tissue** that surrounds the sciatic nerve where it exits the greater sciatic notch in the buttocks muscles is relieved by **RUTA**.

This demonstrates once again the specificity of homeopathic medicine. There is not just one remedy for every person who suffers with sciatica. Understanding how the injury happened, the nature of the pain, and which specific tissues are involved is necessary to choose the correct remedy. In most cases, taking **ARNICA** first not only brings pain relief, but it may also prevent further injury. If **numbness**, **tingling**, or **shooting pain** persists, taking **HYPERICUM** and **ARNICA** together every 2 to 3 hours heals the tissues and can prevent chronic pain. If the tissues are tender to the touch and

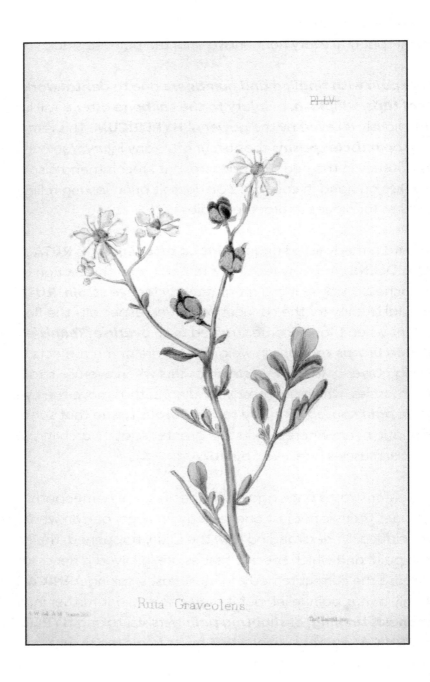

Pl. LV.

Ruta Graveolens.

movement makes the pain better, **RUTA** may also be added to the mix. Giving one remedy at a time and observing what happens is the key, rather than just taking all three remedies blindly from the very beginning. By paying attention to how you feel after you take each remedy, you can gain insight into the nature of the injury. *Chronic sciatic pain* that has lasted for months or even years requires consultation with a professional homeopath.

RUTA is also useful for *injuries to the periosteum*, which is the thin covering of the bones. *Nodules* that form on the front of the legs after knocking your shins repeatedly on the coffee table can be healed with the help of **RUTA.** Tiny microfractures in the periosteum of the shinbones in runners, known as *shin splints,* are another kind of injury where **RUTA** works its magic.

Bell's palsy is a weakness or paralysis of the muscles of one side of the face, usually due to *injury to the facial nerve*. The affected side of the face will droop as we often see in people who have suffered a stroke. However, unlike stroke, the injury is localized to the nerve that supplies the muscles of the face. **CAUSTICUM** is one of the most helpful remedies for this condition, especially when the total symptom picture fits the remedy. **CAUSTICUM** is a remedy for people who have a keen *sense of fairness* and they cannot stand to see anyone treated unjustly.

A number of years ago, a prominent consumer activist was flying across the country and fell asleep with his cheek pressed against the cold window of the airplane. When he awakened, he had Bell's palsy; the facial nerve that innervates his cheek muscle was temporarily injured and that side of his face drooped. **CAUSTICUM** is the remedy he needed at the time.

Hearing this story from my first homeopathy teacher forever
embedded in my memory the relationship between **Bell's palsy**
and **issues of justice.** I certainly didn't learn there was such a
correlation in my neurology courses in medical school. But over the
years, I have had several occasions to use **CAUSTICUM** for patients
with **Bell's palsy**. Inevitably when **CAUSTICUM** was the correct
remedy, each of the patients had a particular cause they were
active in supporting.

When I ask new patients whether they have ever used homeopathic
remedies, most of them tell me that they have used **ARNICA** in the
past for some type of injury. **ARNICA MONTANA** is the quintessential
trauma remedy and the first one to reach for in case of **injury of
any kind** to any part of the body, internal or external. **ARNICA** heals
tissue damage caused by **falls, sprains, accidents, or heart attacks**
if it is given promptly and in frequent doses.

Taking **ARNICA** after a fall can **prevent massive bruising** as we saw
in the case of my patient who suffered a straddle injury from falling
into a swimming pool. For **minor muscle pain or soreness** from too
many push-ups or miles pounding on the treadmill at the gym, the
30c potency repeated every few hours should suffice.

But for more severe injuries such as **fractured bones, head trauma,**
or **whiplash**, the 200c potency is often required. It can be repeated
every hour immediately after injury, depending on the severity of
the wound. Remember, as in the section on head trauma, **NATRUM
SULPHURICUM** is the additional remedy to reach for after **injury to
the head.**

Last summer one of my friends, who is also a client, slipped and
fractured her arm. She immediately started taking **ARNICA** and

RUTA as we headed for the emergency room. She took both remedies every hour while we waited for the X-ray to be taken and the temporary splint to be applied. She never developed any bruising or swelling despite having a clean break of one of the bones in her forearm.

Once the X-ray showed that the bone was not displaced, we added **SYMPHYTUM OFFICINALE** to help the bone to heal. She continued all three remedies two to three times a day until a repeat X-ray showed the fracture was completely healed. Remember to ***never start SYMPHYTUM until an X-ray shows that the bone is properly set.*** **SYMPHYTUM** is a powerful bone knitter and being certain the bone is properly aligned before taking it ensures the bone heals in the correct anatomical position.

In cases where a ***fracture has failed to heal,*** even after taking **SYMPHYTUM,** adding **CALCAREA PHOSPHORICUM**, the remedy used for ***growing pains in children***, will often stimulate the bone to heal completely. During the 19th century, **CALC PHOS** was used for the treatment of ***rickets*** (a disease of childhood that results in soft or weak bones due to a vitamin D deficiency) because of its propensity to stimulate bone growth, like **SYMPHYTUM**.

Obviously, in more severe cases of trauma such as ***gunshot wounds*** or ***stabbings***, **ARNICA** is just one of the remedies that should be given on the way to the hospital. **LEDUM PALUSTRE,** the main remedy for ***puncture wounds***, and **CALENDULA** or **HAMAMELIS** for ***bleeding*** (depending on the situation), are also part of the complement of remedies used for ***severe trauma***. In cases where there is extreme blood loss requiring a transfusion, **CHINA OFFICINALIS** is often needed to treat the extreme ***fatigue that often accompanies massive blood loss.*** However, treating such extreme cases requires professional homeopathic consultation. But having these remedies on hand is vital in cases of trauma. It doesn't help to have the advice of a homeopath in these cases if you don't have the remedies required.

Simple **sprains** are a perfect setting for the healing power of homeopathic remedies. Besides **RUTA GRAVEOLENS**, the other remedy that is especially helpful for injuries to the muscles and tendons surrounding a joint is **RHUS TOXICODENDRON**. You may recall that this is one of the remedies used for **shingles** or other **herpes infections**. **RHUS TOX** is the homeopathic preparation of poison oak and therefore has a particular action on the skin. But it is especially helpful after injuries to the extremities.

The hallmark symptoms of **RHUS TOX** are **stiffness on waking** in the morning that gets **better once you start to move** around. However, **overexertion** will bring the pain and stiffness back. When treating sprains of any kind, I usually recommend taking **RUTA** 30c every few hours first. If **stiffness or pain** persists, add **RHUS TOX** 30c and take them together every 3 to 4 hours. These two remedies should be in the gym bag of every weekend warrior for the relief they bring to sore limbs. Taking these remedies often precludes having to take ibuprofen or aspirin after injuries or overexertion.

As learned in the section on joint pain, **BRYONIA** is the remedy that has a contrasting symptom picture to **RHUS TOX;** pain that is **worse with any motion** indicates the Vital Force is calling for **BRYONIA**, not **RHUS TOX. BRYONIA** is also the remedy to consider **when ARNICA fails** to bring relief after injuries to any joint and movement of any kind is almost impossible due to pain.

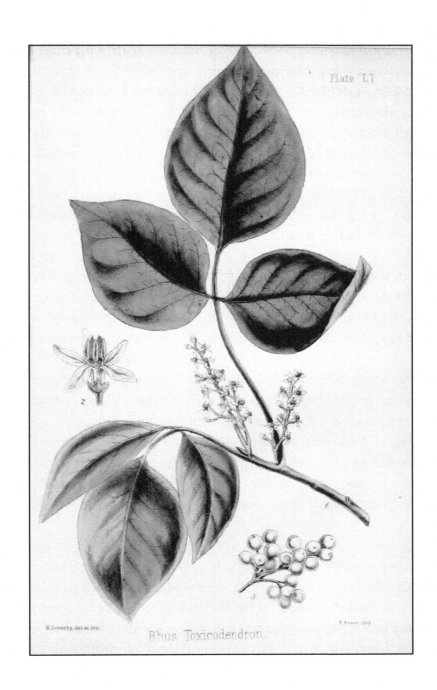

Plate LI

2

1

3

B. Sowerby del et lith.

P. Reeve imp.

Rhus Toxicodendron.

CALCAREA FLUORICA is one of the over-the-counter remedies that's helpful for people who are constantly *spraining their ankles*. *Easy dislocation of the joints* is another symptom that calls for **CALCAREA FLUORICA,** also called **CALCAREA FLUORATA.** When I was a medical student on the orthopedics service at the county hospital, one of my patients was a prisoner brought over from the jail. He could easily pop his shoulder out of its socket, which he did at will in order to come to the hospital for pain medications and better food. (The food in the jail must have been *really* bad because it wasn't that great in the hospital either.) I'm sure this remedy could have helped him but clearly that wasn't his desire.

Instead, the court ordered him to have a Barlow's procedure: the head of the biceps tendon is moved from the arm and reattached across the shoulder joint to prevent the head of the femur from dislocating. The other thing I remember about that case were the two burly prison guards dressed in barely fitting surgical scrubs who handcuffed him to the table and stood right outside the door during the entire case. When I asked them why they used handcuffs on someone who would soon be completely unconscious, they said, "You'll see." Sure enough, when the prisoner awakened from anesthesia, he came up swinging and the guards had to physically restrain him to keep him from tearing his newly repaired shoulder. Clearly a homeopathic remedy alone wasn't going to work in that case.

One other remedy that is helpful in a very specific type of trauma is **SILICA**. This remedy was discussed earlier in regard to migraine headaches. **SILICA**, which is made from flint, has the unique ability to *dislodge foreign objects.* A splinter, a BB, or a piece of shrapnel stuck below the surface of the skin can be extruded using **SILICA**.

A number of years ago, one of my patients brought her teenaged daughter to see me for help with heavy, irregular menstrual periods. As I took her history, she told me that she had been injured in a car accident where the window shattered and sprayed her face with dozens of tiny shards of glass that had become embedded in her skin. When I examined her, I could feel multiple little bumps right under the surface of her skin along the right side of her cheek and jaw.

I started her on **SILICA** 30c twice daily and scheduled her to return for a follow-up visit in 6 weeks. Sure enough, she reported that she would wake up with tiny slivers of glass on her pillow every morning. It took almost a year but eventually all the glass came out of her face, painlessly, as we gradually increased the potency every month or so. The other added benefit was her menses became regular and the flow was no longer heavy. A word of caution about **SILICA.** Because of its power to extrude a foreign body, this is *not* the remedy to use in people with silicone chin, breast, or butt implants. I would not use it in patients with artificial joints for the same reason.

SURGICAL REMEDIES

Surgery is often called controlled trauma and for good reason. I recommended homeopathic remedies for all my patients undergoing surgery and I provided them with a list of the remedies to bring to the hospital. In their admission orders to the hospital I included, "patient may take their own homeopathic remedies from home." I never encountered any difficulties with the hospital administration because my patients took remedies while in house.

I found over the years that taking homeopathic remedies helped my patients have less bleeding, less bruising, and they needed less pain medication. I gave up using prophylactic antibiotics for routine surgeries years ago, once I became a homeopath. The following are the remedies that I routinely used for all my surgical patients. They don't interfere with any of the medications that your surgeon or other health care practitioner may prescribe for you. You may wish to discuss taking homeopathic remedies with your surgeon. However, be prepared if the response you receive is negative. We don't learn about homeopathy in conventional medical school and most doctors don't know the first thing about what it is or how to use homeopathic remedies properly. Fear of the unknown therefore leads most doctors to dismiss homeopathy and recommend you not take them. However, the remedies are safe to take and the ones I recommend are readily available over the counter in most natural food stores.

ARNICA MONTANA is, of course, the queen of trauma remedies, and it's the first one to take if you are having surgery of any kind, especially *cosmetic surgery*. Its power in *preventing bruising* has made it a favorite of most plastic surgeons and is routinely recommended for patients having facelifts or other procedures where there is extensive manipulation of soft tissue that is rich in small blood vessels and prone to easy bruising. You can take one dose of the 30c potency under the tongue on your way to the hospital, although your doctor may have instructed you not to take anything by mouth. One pellet under the tongue will not put you at risk of choking or vomiting.

After the surgery, take the 30c potency every 8 hours or three times a day until the incision is completely healed. In most cases, this prevents all bruising except for a little yellow discoloration of the skin about 10 days postoperatively, which is the normal healing time for a full-blown bruise. But you will have avoided the painful purple discoloration that is common after any trauma, controlled or otherwise.

As learned in the section on bladder infections, **STAPHYSAGRIA** is the remedy to have on hand not only for full-blown *infections of the bladder* but also for the pain that can come from having a urinary catheter inserted in the bladder during, and in some cases remaining after, surgery. Besides urinary tract pain, **STAPHYSAGRIA** is helpful for people who have *postoperative pain that persists* longer than usual. Many times, this remedy helped my patients who were still complaining of intense pain several weeks after surgery when the need for pain medications should have been diminished. **STAPHYSAGRIA** is also helpful for *preventing infection at the site of the incision.*

CALENDULA, a remedy for *burns*, is also a wonderful remedy for *preventing wound infections.* It helps the skin heal after surgery or any penetrating wounds, such as *stab* or *gunshot wounds*, especially where there is a high risk of infection. In the days before antibiotics, homeopaths used this remedy to prevent *pyemia*, an abscess of the lung, as well as *gangrene*. In cases of *diabetic ulcers,* **MRSA** (methicillin-resistant *Staphylococcus aureus* infections), or *bedsores* where gangrene is a real threat and antibiotics have failed to work, **CALENDULA** could save a life or a limb as it has in millions of cases treated homeopathically throughout the world in the last 250 years.

CALENDULA is especially helpful in cases of *bleeding* where there is *oozing from the small blood vessels.* Taken with **ARNICA** after tooth extraction, **CALENDULA** can prevent *dry socket*, a painful condition where the blood clot that normally forms in the jaw at the site of the extraction gets dislodged. This exposes the nerve and the bone to air, fluid, and food and can be very painful. However, taking **ARNICA** and **CALENDULA** in the 30c potency every 8 hours after tooth extraction will prevent this painful complication.

CALENDULA is available over the counter only in a topical cream or gel. However, when using it to stop bleeding or prevent infection, the higher potencies of 30c or even 200c are necessary. You can order these online from a homeopathic pharmacy in single doses or as part of a home emergency kit. (See resources.)

HAMAMELIS is the other remedy that is helpful in stopping bleeding in postoperative patients. You will recall this is the remedy I used in my two patients who had postoperative bleeding from faulty sutures that started to dissolve too soon. **HAMAMELIS** is also helpful for stopping *excessive menstrual bleeding* or *bleeding due to fibroid tumors.* The 30c potency, repeated every few hours, is often strong enough to *stop postoperative bleeding, or oozing.* On rare occasions, I have had to use the 200c for women with bleeding fibroids when the 30c potency didn't hold.

Swelling is a common problem after injury to the soft tissues and **APIS** is the remedy that can bring substantial relief and help decrease the need for pain medication. Taking the 30c potency every few hours is usually sufficient. However, in cases of extensive trauma after accidents or surgery, the 200c potency is often required.

As in any acute situation treated homeopathically, it's best to continue to take the trauma remedies regularly until the injury or surgical incision is completely healed. You can decrease the frequency of the remedy gradually as your recovery progresses. A rough rule of thumb is to continue to take the remedies at least once a day for a few days after *all* of your symptoms have resolved.

Another important part of recovering from surgery is **removing the effects of general anesthesia**. Multiple medications are required to keep you safely unconscious and immobile during surgery. These drugs are essentially controlled toxins and without them modern surgery would be impossible. These medications are delivered either as inhaled gases, intravenously, or injected locally into the skin. No matter how they are delivered, they must still be metabolized by your liver and kidneys, which are elegantly designed to do just that.

In cases where you awaken from anesthesia feeling like you've been on a weekend-long bender in Las Vegas, **NUX VOMICA** is just what your doctor would order if he or she were homeopathically inclined. I found that well over 50% of my surgical patients needed **NUX VOMICA** to help them recover from anesthesia. In most cases, taking the 30c potency once or twice a day for the first few days after surgery does the trick. You'll recall that this is the first remedy to consider for a **hangover** because of its great detoxifying powers.

For nausea and/or vomiting that persist after anesthesia, there are homeopathic remedies that can be given in lieu of more drugs. **PHOSPHORUS** is indicated in cases of *prolonged vomiting after anesthesia.* **PHOSPHORUS** is the remedy to consider when vomiting occurs as soon as whatever you drink becomes warm in the stomach. **ARSENICUM ALBUM** is the remedy to take when the *vomiting occurs immediately after drinking*.

TRAVEL

Although we have covered the following remedies in detail elsewhere in the book, I have grouped them together to make it easier for you to include them in your travel kit. In most cases, the 30c potency will be sufficient. However, I would also get the 200c potency of **ARNICA** if your local health food store carries it. There are a few remedies that you will need to order from an online homeopathic pharmacy.

We are certainly aware of, or unfortunately experience ourselves, the trauma caused by car accidents, physical assaults, or thefts and robberies. **ACONITUM NAPELLUS** is the remedy to take immediately after something traumatic happens; it's the first remedy to reach for in cases of *shock,* whether physical, mental, or emotional. **ACONITE** is indicated in frightful situations where *death or severe injury* is threatened. Getting robbed at gunpoint can definitely put you in a *state of fear* that is one of the keynote symptoms calling for **ACONITE.** Taking the 30c potency once or twice a day until the panic passes can spare you the long-term effects of shock such as *posttraumatic stress disorder.*

APIS MELLIFICA earns inclusion in your travel kit for its amazing ability to *reduce swelling* from any cause. Soft tissue injury from trauma, insect stings, or blood clots in the legs from sitting in an airplane for many hours can all produce swelling. It may be necessary to repeat the remedy every hour or so until the swelling subsides. In cases of blood clots, the best treatment is to prevent them in the first place by moving the legs or getting up and walking every hour or so on long flights. **APIS** is especially helpful when the *tissues are red, hot, and tender to the touch as well as swollen.* **LEDUM PALUSTRE** is the first remedy to take for any sting, bite, or puncture wound, including bee stings. If swelling persists or develops after a sting despite taking several doses of **LEDUM** over a few hours, it's time to add **APIS** to the mix. Taking both **LEDUM** and **APIS** together after a serious bite or puncture when the *tissues are red*, *hot*, and *swollen* helps prevent infection and speeds healing.

ARGENTUM NITRICUM and **GELSEMIUM SEMPERVIRENS** are two remedies that are helpful for nervous travelers. Both are discussed in depth in the section on fear of flying, and you may want to review that section to help you choose which remedy to take if you get nervous before traveling. It's wise to have both with you when you travel if you or your fellow travelers tend to be anxious flyers.

ARNICA MONTANA, the premier remedy for trauma, is an essential part of any first aid kit. It's helpful for sore feet and muscles after you've been hiking or tramping through museums for hours at a time. Taking the 30c potency along with a hot Epsom salt bath before bedtime works better than ibuprofen or acetaminophen, in my experience, and is easier on your liver and kidneys.

I never travel anywhere without **ARSENICUM ALBUM**, the quintessential remedy for food poisoning. For more detail on how to use this vacation-saving remedy, review the section on food poisoning. It has personally saved me four trips to the hospital over the years when I encountered tainted food while traveling.

BELLADONNA is a must-have remedy if you're traveling with children or plan to spend long periods of time in the sun. *Sudden onset of a high fever* from infection or from *sunstroke*, especially if the **face is red** or **flushed**, is the perfect setting for **BELLADONNA**. I have seen it bring the temperature down from well over 102°F to 98.6°F in under 20 minutes. If the fever begins to climb back up, you can repeat the dose every 15 to 20 minutes. Determining the underlying cause of the fever is paramount and may require professional attention.

BRYONIA is a handy remedy to have when you travel for its ability to relieve pain after injury or overexertion that's **worse with motion.** It's the first remedy to think of for **acute appendicitis** when the slightest touch or jarring brings excruciating pain. Taking the 30c potency every 20 to 30 minutes on the way to the hospital can begin to calm an inflamed belly. Under the proper guidance of a well-trained homeopath, it can even preclude the need for surgery. Obviously, do not try this at home if you have not had years of professional homeopathic training and experience.

CALENDULA earns its place in your travel kit for several reasons. It can **stop bleeding, heal burns,** and **prevent infection after cuts or scrapes to the skin.** One of my teachers used it to successfully treat his father in the midst of a stroke caused by bleeding in the brain. As in any emergency or acute situation, the dose and frequency of the remedy needs to match the intensity of the symptoms. Severe symptoms require frequent dosing and sometimes a higher potency. Start with the 30c potency every few hours and, if the relief doesn't last, go up to the 200c.

CARBO VEGETABILIS is another helpful travel remedy because of its power to heal respiratory troubles. The hallmark symptom that calls for **CARBO VEG** is **shortness of breath,** or **dyspnea.** Dyspnea can occur as a result of bronchitis or pneumonia. Hiking at high altitude can also trigger shortness of breath but there's a remedy for preventing altitude sickness that we'll meet in a moment. We've already covered its use at the deathbed but hopefully you won't have occasion to use it for that while you're on vacation!

If you have ever hiked Machu Picchu in Peru, perhaps your travel guide offered you a cup of tea brewed from coca leaves. Chewing coca leaf has long been used by indigenous people in South America for its ability to increase stamina and treat the symptoms of altitude sickness. My brother in law JP loves to travel and to ski. But until he learned about **COCCINELLA**, altitude sickness limited him to skiing mountains well under 9,000 feet. **COCCINELLA** is the code name for a homeopathic preparation made from the coca leaf—it is available only by prescription from a homeopathic practitioner. Not only does it allow JP to come to Colorado to ski, it also helped one of his colleagues successfully climb Mt. Kilimanjaro last year after a previous attempt had failed due to altitude sickness.

One of my long-term patients, Ann, is a very active person who enjoys hiking and biking along with working out with a trainer twice a week. Her base camp is Phoenix, Arizona, at an altitude of 1,086 feet, but she experienced altitude sickness on a hiking trip to Peru—thankfully, she had her travel kit of remedies with her.

As a treat, I planned a trip to the Sacred Valley in Peru, traveling roughly 16 hours with two flights so I could get to the area as quickly as possible and enjoy every moment of my vacation. The elevation at Cusco where I stayed was 11,200 feet. Aware of dehydration on the flights and the possible exacerbation of altitude sickness, I tried to increase my water intake in flight. Upon landing and unpacking at the hotel, I took a quick shower and planned on getting a walk in as well as some food before the sun descended and the cold set in. Usually enjoying plenty of energy, I found that I was moving more slowly than normal. But at that point, I figured it was probably a combination of jetlag, dehydration, and altitude. I took a dosage of **COCCINELLA** 30c. Leaving the hotel, I was in awe of the Inca walls, cathedrals, women in traditional colorful skirts with llamas or lambs, alpaca knit stores, and the endless hawkers of massages. But the sun was almost down, and the temperature was plummeting, so I turned back around to go get a jacket from the hotel. I'd probably been out walking for roughly an hour, and as I made my way back to the hotel lobby, I realized that I really didn't have the energy to go out again. In fact, a tremendous headache was enveloping my head. The hotel had a restaurant, so I decided to just eat there and then turn in early. As I perused the menu, I realized I didn't have much of an interest in trying any of the native food. This was sort of shocking as I love new foods and part of my love of traveling is to try new cuisine, which I'd been really looking forward to on this trip.

Sacrificing a meal out of my limited time seemed like blasphemy, but, alas, a chicken sandwich was the only thing that sounded reasonable. As I waited for the order, complete exhaustion was taking over. I laid my head on the table, not really caring what anyone around might be thinking. My head was just too heavy and hurt to move. When the sandwich arrived, I just couldn't stomach eating it. The only thing that held any interest were the French fries. To have traveled all this way, and have French fries! I ate some of them, but my stomach wasn't feeling very settled. I asked for the sandwich to be wrapped up. It felt like years before the waiter returned with the sandwich and bill.

Back in my hotel room, I lay down on one of the two beds. My head was pounding, I didn't want to move, and just wanted to keep my eyes closed. I forced myself up to get another dosage of **COCCINELLA**. The headache pain was awful. I laid down again, and had thoughts of dying in the hotel room, my suitcase unpacked hastily and stuff spread all over the other bed. I thought, "Wow, who is going to be able to get that all packed and get my body out of the country and back home?"

Through the night, I forced myself to get up, drink water. I kept up the 30c dosage every couple of hours. By morning, I was able to go to breakfast. I was short of breath, as that altitude takes time to acclimate to, but I passed by another traveler in the lobby area who was unable to control the nausea sadly. Fortunately, I only had the severe headache and downtime for that first evening. I was able to continue my explorations, and continued taking 30c dosages every 4 hours for the first few days of the trip.

CINCHONA OFFICINALIS, or CHINA, is an essential part of any traveler's kit for its ability to treat traveler's diarrhea. You'll recall from earlier discussion that it's especially helpful for **diarrhea** that occurs **after drinking bad water or eating unclean fruit.** **Abdominal bloating** and **gas** and a **feeling of being wiped out** are all key symptoms that **CHINA** will relieve.

The other must-have remedy for traveler's diarrhea is **PODOPHYLLUM**. **Yellowish-green diarrhea** that comes out in a **sudden gush without pain** or cramping calls for **PODOPHYLLUM**. Unlike cases where **CHINA** is the needed remedy, extreme fatigue or weakness isn't part of the symptom picture of **PODOPHYLLUM**.

Nothing ruins a vacation quite like motion sickness. No one wants to be vomiting in the head while their friends and family are up on deck enjoying the sunshine and catching lots of fish. As we discussed in the section on motion sickness, **COCCULUS** and **TABACUM** are the

165

two main remedies to have when you travel if you're prone to this thrill-killing ailment.

COCCULUS is the remedy to reach for when *headache* comes along with the *nausea and vomiting*. *Weakness or fatigue* and *intolerance to cold air* are key symptoms indicating **COCCULUS** is the right choice. In contrast, **TABACUM** patients crave fresh, cool air and feel better if they can get outside of a stuffy stateroom or car. There's a lot of *spitting of saliva* that's part of the **TABACUM** symptom picture also. (See the section on motion sickness for a more detailed discussion on how to choose between these two remedies.)

COFFEA CRUDA is helpful to have on hand when you're traveling due to its ability to help with *insomnia*. When an overactive mind precludes sleep, **COFFEA CRUDA** 30c before bedtime will often quiet the mind and bring on restful sleep. You can repeat it if you awaken during the night; usually there's no morning drowsiness that is a frequent side effect of pharmaceutical sleep medications.

Jet lag due to travel across time zones can often disrupt your normal sleep schedule, leaving you wide awake in the middle of the night and then falling asleep on the tour bus the next afternoon. In general, I'm not a big fan of combination products that contain more than one homeopathic remedy. In my opinion, they work more like a shotgun than a laser beam and, in general, I recommend single-dose remedies that are specific for your symptoms and the circumstances that elicited them. The one exception I usually make is "No-Jet-Lag" made by Miers Laboratories in New Zealand. It contains a combination of five remedies in the 30c potency and is readily available throughout the world in airports, travel stores, and health food stores. Visit their website at www.nojetlag.com.

for more information on where to get it and how to take it. Simple instructions are also provided on the box.

Note: They claim that their product is manufactured in such a way that it is impervious to X-rays. I'm not sure how this can be so, but to play it safe I would *not* put the remedy through the X-ray scanner nor pack it in your checked luggage. (See Chapter One for a reminder on how to safely get your remedies through airport security.)

In the section on bone pain, we learned about one of my favorite remedies, **EUPATORIUM PERFOLIATUM**. I've included it in the list of travel remedies because of its ability to **relieve bone pain** and high fever that occur with some exotic infections like **malaria** and **dengue fever**. These conditions occur in tropical locations and are transmitted by mosquitoes. Sleeping under mosquito netting when camping in tropical areas is crucial to prevent being bitten. The main symptom that calls for **EUPATORIUM** in these circumstances is **severe pain deep in the long bones** of the extremities. It may be necessary to repeat the remedy every 30 to 60 minutes for several hours to bring relief. I would start with the 30c potency and continue as long as it brings relief. If the pain returns, you may need the 200c potency so it's a good idea to be sure to include both potencies in your travel kit.

As discussed in the section on colds, **FERRUM PHOSPHORICUM** is the remedy to take at the **beginning stages of any inflammatory condition** such as a **cold**, **the flu**, or **an ear infection**. The symptom picture can include a sore or scratchy throat, headache, nasal congestion, body aches, or ear pain. The distinguishing feature of **FERRUM PHOS** is that the symptoms come on slowly over a day or two.

In cases where cold or flu symptoms *come on suddenly*, especially after exposure to cold or *windy weather*, **ACONITUM NAPELLUS** is usually the remedy that brings relief. In either case, take the appropriate remedy in the 30c potency every 4 to 6 hours. As your symptoms abate, slowly decrease the frequency of the remedy but don't stop the remedy abruptly. Taking the remedy at least once a day for 3 days after all your symptoms are gone will help prevent a relapse.

GELSEMIUM SEMPERVIRENS belongs in every traveler's kit especially for those who are nervous fliers. In addition to its ability to relieve *anxiety before a trip*, **GELSEMIUM** is also a powerful remedy for the *flu*. *Weakness*, *body aches*, and *anxiety* about being sick, especially when you're away from home, are common symptoms that call for **GELSEMIUM**. (For a more detailed discussion, see the sections on anxiety and flu.)

HAMAMELIS is included in the previous discussions on bleeding. Made from witch hazel, **HAMAMELIS** has an amazing ability to stop *bleeding*, especially oozing from small blood vessels. Cuts or scrapes that continue to bleed despite a pressure bandage but are not deep enough to require stitches are a perfect setting for **HAMAMELIS**.

As discussed earlier, **CALENDULA** is the other remedy to consider for bleeding. The difference between the two is that **CALENDULA** is especially helpful in situations where the risk of infection is high. A cut or abrasion that occurs in less than hygienic circumstances is a good time to add **CALENDULA**, either applied as an ointment or taken in pellet form in the 30c potency.

Remember, the hiking geriatrician with sciatic pain? The remedy he needed to treat the sciatica he developed after hiking Camelback Mountain in Phoenix was **HYPERICUM**. This remedy is a miracle worker when it comes to pain from injury to areas of the body that are especially sensitive due to their high concentration of nerve endings. ***Shooting pain with numbness or tingling*** from injury to any nerve is a clear call for **HYPERICUM**. Hikers and climbers should never leave home without **HYPERICUM** and **ARNICA**, too.

IPECACUANHA earns its place in the roster of travel remedies for its ability to relieve ***nausea that doesn't go away even after vomiting***. It's helpful for ***motion sickness*** or in cases of **food poisoning** where the nausea and vomiting persist despite taking **ARSENICUM ALBUM**.

LEDUM PALUSTRE belongs in your travel kit, especially if you are going to places beloved by biting and stinging creatures. It's the remedy to take for ***bee and wasp stings*** as well as ***mosquito bites***. Any injury involving a ***puncture*** is the perfect setting for **LEDUM**. It can prevent tetanus infection as well.

NUX VOMICA belongs in every party planner's bag; nothing treats a hangover better than **NUX VOMICA** in the 30c potency. For severe cases, take the remedy every hour until the headache, nausea, and heartburn begin to subside. Adequate fluids, extra vitamin C, and a dose of **NUX VOMICA** before bedtime after a night of revelry can prevent a hangover and help you be ready for the next day's itinerary.

The remedy **RHUS TOXICODENDRON** was introduced earlier in the discussion about remedies for ***herpes***, ***shingles***, and ***arthritis***. Made from poison oak, **RHUS TOX** is the first remedy to reach for if you develop a blistery rash after stepping in poison ivy, poison oak, or poison sumac.

URTICA URENS, made from stinging nettle, is the other remedy to have on hand in cases of hives with ***intense itching***. Unlike the **RHUS TOX** rash, the skin eruptions are not vesicular or blistered. Red ***raised welts*** that make you want to scratch to the point of bleeding are relieved with **URTICA URENS**.

STAPHYSAGRIA and **CANTHARIS VULGARIS** are must-have remedies for first or second time honeymooners for their ability to treat ***urinary tract infections*** without antibiotics. For a more thorough discussion on how to choose between these two remedies, see the section on bladder infections.

In summary, here's a list of the remedies that you should carry with you when you travel. Remember to always ask the TSA agent to hand check your remedies. Remedies work energetically, not biochemically, so putting them through the X-ray machine at the airport completely annihilates their healing powers.

ACONITUM NAPELLUS
APIS MELLIFICA
ARGENTUM NITRICUM
ARNICA MONTANA
ARSENICUM ALBUM
BELLADONNA
BRYONIA ALBA
CALENDULA OFFICINALIS
CARBO VEGETABILIS
COCCINELLA (COCA LEAF)
CINCHONA OFFICINALIS (CHINA)

COCCULUS INDICUS
COFFEA CRUDA
EUPATORIUM PERFOLIATUM
FERRUM PHOSPHORICUM
GELSEMIUM SEMPERVIRENS
HAMAMELIS OCCIDENTALIS
HYPERICUM PERFORATUM
IPECACUANHA
LEDUM PALUSTRE
NUX VOMICA
PODOPHYLLUM PELTATUM
RHUS TOXICODENDRON
STAPHYSAGRIA
TABACUM
URTICA URENS

Chapter 3
What's Next?
———— ༄ ————

Hopefully you have enjoyed this introduction to the world of homeopathic medicine and are eager to give it a try. If you follow the guidelines laid out for you throughout the book, I think you will be pleasantly surprised at the healing power that you can harness to help yourself and your family. By simply "matching" the mental, emotional, and physical symptoms of your illness with the symptom picture of the appropriate remedy, you can hasten your recovery from illness or injury and, in many cases, avoid having to go to the doctor.

There is something very empowering in being able to take charge of your own health care. Using homeopathic remedies allows you to ease suffering for yourself and your family. Each time you choose a remedy instead of a pharmaceutical drug, you are stimulating your body's innate ability to heal itself. With each illness treated successfully, you actually become healthier as the remedy peels off another layer of energetic "dis-ease" accumulated from living in our overstimulated and sometimes toxic environment.

Of course, you must trust yourself enough to make good decisions. If you aren't sure about the remedy you have chosen, you can always consult a professional homeopath for help. Choosing a good homeopath can be as easy or as difficult as choosing a good pediatrician or orthopedic surgeon, but with an additional wrinkle. The training programs and certification boards for homeopathy are not as standardized as they are for conventional medicine. There are many excellent homeopaths who are neither medical doctors nor naturopathic physicians but have devoted their lives to the study of homeopathy.

When choosing a homeopath, I suggest interviewing them either over the phone or in person before you become a client. If that is not available, perhaps they have a website that will give you information about their background and training. It is best to choose a homeopathic practitioner, either lay or professional, who has been studying and working primarily as a homeopath for a minimum of ten years, in my opinion. Although there are practitioners who have also trained in other modalities such as herbal medicine, the homeopaths with the highest accuracy in recommending the correct remedy are those who devote the majority of their study and practice exclusively to the homeopathic modality.

There are over 5,000 remedies available to treat virtually every illness known to humanity. Just taking an online course is not enough training to acquire the skill and expertise required to become a good homeopath. Seeing actual clients daily for many years, initially under the supervision of an experienced practitioner, is necessary to master the complex art and science of homeopathy. Any skilled and well-qualified homeopath will be happy to share their credentials with you before you decide to become a client.

Resources

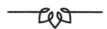

HOMEOPATHIC PHARMACIES

Boiron
6 Campus Boulevard
Newtown Square, PA 19073
(800) 264 7661
www.boironusa.com

Hahnemann Laboratories, Inc.
Mail Order Pharmacy
San Rafael, CA 94901
(888) 427 6422
www.hahnemannlabs.com

Natural Health Supply
6410 Avenida Christina
Santa Fe, NM 87507
www.a2zhomeopathy.com

Phoenix Medicinary
(Formerly American Medical College of Homeopathy Medicinary)
301 E. Bethany Home Rd, Ste A-135
Phoenix, AZ 85012
www.phoenixmedicinary.com

Santa Monica Homeopathic Pharmacy
629 Broadway
Santa Monica, CA 90401
www.smhomeopathic.com

Southwest College of Naturopathic Medicine Medicinary
2152 E. Broadway Rd
Tempe, AZ 85282
480 970 0001
www.patients.scnm.edu/services/scnm-medicinary

Washington Homeopathic Products
260 J R Hawvermale Way
Berkeley Springs, WV 25411
www.homeopathyworks.com

REFERENCES

Allen, Timothy Field. A Primer of Materia Medica for Practitioners of Homeopathy. Philadelphia: Boericke and Tafel; 1892.

Allen, Timothy Field. The Encyclopedia of Pure Materia Medica: A Record of the Positive Effects of Drugs upon the Healthy Human Organism. New York: Boericke & Tafel; [c1874]-79.

Boenninghausen, Clemens Maria Franz von. A Systematic, Alphabetic Repertory of Homeopathic Remedies [transl. from the 2nd German ed., by C. M. Boger]. Philadelphia: Boericke & Tafel; 1900.

Boericke, William. Materia Medica with Repertory, 9th edition. Santa Rosa, CA: Boericke & Tafel, Inc.; 1927.

Clarke, John Henry. Dictionary of Practical Materia Medica. Vol. I-III. 3rd edition. Sittingbourne, Kent, UK: Homeopathic Book Service; 1991.

Hahnemann, Samuel. The Chronic Diseases, their Peculiar Nature and their Homeopathic Cure [transl. from the 2nd enlarged German ed. of 1835, by Prof. Louis H. Tafel]. Dresden. Germany: Arnoldischen Buchhandlung; 1828.

Hamilton, Edward. The Flora Homeopathic: Illustrations and Descriptions of the Medicinal Plants Used as Homeopathic Remedies, two volumes. London: H. Bailliere, London; 1852 and 1853.

Hering, Constantine: The Guiding Symptoms of our Materia Medica. Philadelphia: Estate of C. Hering; c1879-1891. [Note: Vols. 3-10 completed after the author's death by C.G. Raue, C.B. Knerr, and C. Mohr.]

Idarius, Betty. The Homeopathic Childbirth Manual: A Practical Guide for Labor, Birth and the Immediate Postpartum Period. Ukiah, CA: Idarius Press; 1996.

Kent, James Tyler. Lectures on Homeopathic Materia Medica, 3rd ed. Philadelphia: Boericke & Tafel; 1923.

Kent, James Tyler. Lectures on Homeopathic Philosophy. Berkeley, CA: North Atlantic Books. Homeopathic Educational Services; 1979.

MacRepertory 8.5.2.10 Professional version. Novato, CA: Synergy Homeopathic (formerly Kent Homeopathic Associates); 1986-2016. Murphy, Robin. Nature's Materia Medica, 3rd ed. Toronto, Canada: Narayana Publishers; 2006.

Referenceworks 4.5.3.1 Professional version. Novato, CA Synergy Homeopathic (formerly Kent Homeopathic Associates); 1986-2016.

Van Zandvoort, Roger. The Complete Repertory, ed. Leidschendam, The Netherlands: Institute for Research in Homeopathic Information and Symptomatology; 1996.

Vermeulen, Frans. Concordant Materia Medica. Haarlem, The Netherlands: Emryss Publishers; 2000.

RECOMMENDED READING

Castro, Miranda. Homeopathy for Pregnancy, Birth and Your Baby's First Year. New York: St. Martin's Press; 1993.

Castro, Miranda. The Complete Homeopathy Handbook. New York: St. Martin's Press; 1990.

Clarke, Murray. Natural Baby-Healthy Child. Gold River, CA: Authority Publishing; 2010.

Fry, Kathleen. VITALITY! How to Get It and Keep It: A Homeopath's Guide to Vibrant Health Without Drugs. Boulder, CO: Collette Avenue Press; 2013.

Northrup, Christiane. Women's Bodies, Women's Wisdom, (Revised Edition): Creating Physical and Emotional Health and Healing. New York: Bantam Books; 2010.

Perlmutter, David, with Kristin Loberg. Grain Brain: The Surprising Truth About Wheat, Carb and Sugar-Your Brain's Silent Killers. Boston: Little, Brown and Company; 2013.

Perlmutter, David, and Kristin Loberg. The Grain Brain Whole Life Plan: Boost Brain Performance, Lose Weight and Achieve Optimal Health. Boston: Little, Brown and Company; 2016.

About the Author

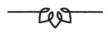

Dr. Fry has been an obstetrician/gynecologist and a homeopath for more than 25 years. She integrated both forms of medicine into her medical practice in Scottsdale, Arizona until 2012, and she now lives in Boulder, Colorado with her family. Her practice is dedicated solely to homeopathy and holistic medicine. She is available for private consultations via Skype, telephone, and in person by arrangement.

drkathi@drkathifry.com
www.drkathifry.com
(480) 695 1383
kathleen.fry180 via Skype

Index

Belladonna
    for Cheyne-Stokes breathing, 32
    for common cold, 8
    for conjunctivitis, 54
    for ear infection, 49–51
    for fever, 57–58
    for headache, 66–68
    for menopausal hot flashes, 104–5
    for menstrual cramps, 120
    for postpartum afterpains, 120
    for restless sleep, 95–96
    as right-sided remedy, 49–50
    for sunstroke, 67–68, 161–62
    for travel, 161–62
Bell's palsy, 149–50
Birth. See Childbirth
Bites, insect, 91–94, 161, 169
Bitter cucumber, 44
Black cohosh, 123. See also Cimicifuga racemosa
Bladder incontinence, 20
Bladder infections, 21–25
    Cantharis for, 22, 170
    individualized remedies for, 22
    Staphysagria for, 22–24, 129, 170
    test kit for, 24–25
    travel remedies for, 170
Bleeding
    Calendula officinalis for, 157–58, 162, 168
    Hamamelis virginiana for, 158, 168
    heavy menstrual, 117, 122–23, 126–28, 158
    in trauma, 151–52
    vicarious menstrual, 126–27
Bleeding hemorrhoids, 90
Blisters, Rhus tox for, 27
Bloating, abdominal, 9, 165
Blood clots, Apis mellifica for, 92–94

Blue cohosh, 121, 123
Boiron, 5, 175
Bone fractures, 30–31, 64, 150–51
Bone pain, 26–30
Bryonia alba for, 27–28
    Eupatorium perfoliatum for, 28–29, 58, 60, 167
    flu and, 26–30, 58, 60
    Gelsemium sempervirens for, 28–29
    Rhus tox for, 26–28
"Bone set," 30
Borax venata, 38
Breast inflammation (mastitis), Phytolacca for, 132–34
Breathing difficulties, 31–33
    Aconite for, 19, 32–33, 34
    Antimonium tartaricum for, 33
    in asthma, 19–20, 31–33
    Belladonna for, 32
    Carbo vegetabilis for, 19–20, 32, 162–63
Broken bones, 30–31, 64, 150–51
Bronchi, 33
Bronchitis, 33–35
    Aconite for, 34
    acute, 33
    Antimonium tartaricum for, 35, 40–41
    Carbo vegetabilis for, 35
    chronic, 33–34
    Drosera rotundifolia for, 35
    Dulcamara for, 35
    Ferrum phosphoricum for, 35
    fever with, 35
    Hepar sulphuris calcarea for, 35
Bruising, 35–37
    Arnica montana for, 35–36, 150, 156–57

Hypericum for, 169
Ipecacuanha for, 169
jet lag in, 166–67
Ledum palustre for, 161, 169
list of remedies for, 170–71
motion sickness in, 136, 142–44, 165–66
Nux vomica for, 169
Podophyllum peltatum for, 165
remedy care and packing in, 6–8, 167
Rhus tox for, 169–70
Staphysagria for, 170
Tabacum for, 142–44, 165–66
Urtica urens for, 170
Traveler's diarrhea, 47–48, 61, 165

U

Ulcer(s)
aphthous, 38
diabetic, 157
pressure (bedsores), 157
Ulcerative colitis, 47
United States Homeopathic Pharmacopoeia, 1
Unrefreshing sleep, 97–100
Upper respiratory tract, 33
Upper respiratory tract infections, 33 -35. See also specific types
Aconite for, 15
Antimonium tartaricum for, 33
Urinary incontinence, 20
Urinary tract infections (UTIs), 21–25
Cantharis for, 22, 170
individualized remedies for, 22
Staphysagria for, 22–24, 129, 170
test kit for, 24–25
travel remedies for, 170

Urticaria (hives), 13–14, 170
Urtica urens, 14, 170
Uterine contractions
Caullophyllum for, 121
Chamomilla vulgaris for, 122
Uterine prolapse, 128–29
pessary for, 129
Sepia for, 128
Staphysagria for, 129
UTIs. See Urinary tract infections

V

Vaccination reactions, Thuja for, 130
Vaccination site pain, 91–92
Vaginal warts, Staphysagria for, 129
Venereal warts
Staphysagria for, 129
Thuja for, 130
Venom, snake, 106. See also Lachesis muta
Vertigo
Arsenicum album and, 61
petroleum and, 144
Vesicular eruptions, Rhus tox for, 27
Vicarious menstruation, 126–27
Vitamin D deficiency, 151
Vomiting
Arsenicum album for, 61
flu and, 59
headaches with, 71–73
Ipecacuanha for, 61–63
menstruation-related, 126
morning sickness, 134–42
postoperative, 159
Vomiting, infant
Ipecacuanha for, 138
Podophyllum peltatum for, 139
Vulvar itching, sulphur for, 130